Living with Your OCPD Partner

A Daily Survival Guide to Setting Boundaries, Finding Peace, and Protecting Your Mental Health in a Controlling Relationship

Lorraine Jace Stark

ISBN: 978-1-7642720-3-2

First Edition

Table of Contents

Preface

You're likely worn down—maybe from yet another argument over something trivial, or from lying awake at night wondering why nothing you do ever feels right.

You're not losing your mind. You're dealing with something specific, challenging, and surprisingly common—but also something that most people, including many therapists, don't fully understand.

This book is written for you—the partner who loves someone with Obsessive-Compulsive Personality Disorder (OCPD) but feels like you're drowning in their need to optimize, control, and improve everything around them. I've written it in plain, straightforward language because you don't need more complexity in your life right now. You need clarity, validation, and practical tools that actually work.

Why I Write This Way

You won't find academic jargon or complicated psychological theories in these pages. Instead, you'll find conversations that sound like real people talking about real problems. I write the way I would speak to a friend who called me at midnight, desperate for someone to understand what they're going through.

This approach isn't accidental. Living with OCPD is complicated enough without having to decode clinical language or sift through theoretical concepts that don't help you handle Tuesday morning's crisis about the "incorrect" way you organized the grocery list. You need information you can use immediately, explained in ways that make sense when your brain is tired and your emotions are running high.

I use contractions because that's how people actually talk. I start sentences with "And" and "But" because that's how thoughts connect in real conversations. I ask you direct questions because I want you to feel like we're having a dialogue, not like you're reading a textbook.

Most importantly, I acknowledge when things are difficult. I don't pretend this is easy work or that following a few simple steps will magically transform your relationship. OCPD creates real challenges that require real strategies, patience, and sometimes difficult decisions. You deserve honest guidance that respects the complexity of what you're facing.

About the People in This Book

Throughout these pages, you'll meet people like Sarah and Mark, Jennifer and David, Lisa and Roberto, and many others. These are composite characters—meaning they're created from patterns I've observed across hundreds of real OCPD relationships, but they don't represent any single person or couple.

I use these composite stories because they illustrate what actually happens in the real world. The woman who reorganizes her husband's filing system while he's at work. The man who researches restaurants for two hours before choosing where to have a simple dinner. The teenager who develops anxiety about homework because nothing ever meets their parent's standards. The partner who stops sharing good news because it always gets analyzed for ways it could have been better.

These patterns repeat across OCPD relationships with remarkable consistency. The details change—different people, different triggers, different coping strategies—but the underlying dynamics are strikingly similar. By creating composite characters, I can show you these patterns clearly without violating anyone's privacy or getting caught up in the unique circumstances that might make one person's story less relevant to your situation.

When you read about Jennifer feeling invisible in her marriage, or David's breakthrough moment when medication helped him recognize his anxiety about imperfection, you're reading about experiences that represent thousands of real people. The names are fictional, but the experiences are authentic representations of what OCPD partners face every day.

What You Can Expect

This book follows a logical progression from understanding what you're dealing with, to developing strategies for managing it, to making informed decisions about your future. But you don't have to read it in order. If you're in crisis, jump to the emergency protocols in Chapter 16. If you're questioning your sanity, start with Chapter 1's explanation of what OCPD really looks like in relationships.

Each chapter builds on previous concepts, but also stands alone enough that you can return to specific sections when you need them. I've included practical tools, worksheets, and step-by-step guides because information without application doesn't change anything.

You'll also find that I don't sugarcoat the challenges or promise easy fixes. OCPD relationships can be deeply rewarding when both partners understand what they're working with and commit to appropriate strategies. They can also be genuinely harmful when perfectionist standards overwhelm a partner's sense of self-worth and autonomy. This book helps you distinguish between workable difficulties and deal-breaker dynamics, while providing tools for both scenarios.

A Personal Note

I want you to know that your experiences are valid. The exhaustion, the confusion, the feeling like you're never quite measuring up—these aren't signs of weakness or oversensitivity. They're normal responses to living with someone whose brain processes efficiency and standards differently than most people.

You're not asking for too much when you want to feel valued for who you are rather than constantly improved. You're not being unreasonable when you need space to make decisions without detailed analysis of better alternatives. You're not giving up too easily if you eventually decide that this dynamic isn't sustainable for your mental health.

This book exists because your wellbeing matters. The strategies, insights, and frameworks in these pages have helped thousands of people create more balanced, satisfying relationships while maintaining their sense of self. Some stayed with their OCPD partners and found ways to build mutual respect and appreciation. Others chose different paths that better supported their long-term happiness.

Both choices can be right, depending on your specific circumstances and what you discover about yourself through this process.

My hope is that by the time you finish this book, you'll feel less alone, more confident in your own judgment, and clearer about what you need to thrive—regardless of what anyone else thinks is the optimal way to live your life.

You deserve relationships that energize rather than exhaust you. Let's figure out how to create that, starting now.

Lorraine Jace Stark

Chapter 1: You're not going crazy

Understanding the most misunderstood personality disorder

Sarah stared at her phone, scrolling through yet another relationship forum at 2 AM. Her husband had criticized her dinner preparation method again—not the taste, mind you, but the exact sequence in which she'd added ingredients. "There's a more efficient way," he'd said, taking over the kitchen with military precision. She'd retreated upstairs, feeling that familiar knot in her stomach.

"I feel like I'm living in a minefield," she typed into the support group chat. "Every day, I wake up wondering what I'll do wrong. He's not cruel or violent, but somehow I feel like I'm disappearing."

The responses flooded in immediately. Dozens of people sharing eerily similar stories. Partners who reorganized their grocery lists. Spouses who had detailed opinions about how towels should be folded. Significant others who turned simple decisions into elaborate research projects.

Sarah wasn't alone. Neither are you.

If you've picked up this book, chances are you're living with someone whose need for order and control has turned your relationship into an exhausting performance. You might feel like you're constantly auditioning for the role of "acceptable partner" and somehow always falling short. The person you love has impossibly high standards—not just for themselves, but for everyone around them, especially you.

Here's what I want you to know right now: **You're not going crazy.** What you're experiencing has a name, and it's not your fault.

The misunderstood disorder hiding in plain sight

Obsessive-Compulsive Personality Disorder, or OCPD, affects between 3-8% of the population (Fineberg et al., 2007). That means millions of people are living with partners who exhibit rigid perfectionism, need excessive control, and struggle to delegate tasks or show flexibility. Yet despite how common it is, OCPD remains one of the most misunderstood mental health conditions.

Unlike many other personality disorders, people with OCPD don't typically seek help. Why would they? In their minds, they're the ones doing everything right. They're organized, responsible, and detail-oriented. If there are problems in the relationship, it must be because their partner isn't trying hard enough to meet reasonable standards.

This creates a particularly painful dynamic for partners. You're left wondering if you really are too messy, too spontaneous, too careless. You second-guess your decisions and find yourself walking on eggshells, trying to anticipate what might trigger the next lecture about "the right way" to do things.

The truth is this: OCPD isn't about having high standards. It's about having impossible ones.

Let me paint you a picture of what OCPD actually looks like in daily life. Your partner doesn't just prefer things done a certain way—they genuinely believe their way is the only logical, efficient, correct way. When you do something differently, they don't see it as a preference issue. They see it as you making an objectively poor choice that needs to be corrected.

This isn't stubbornness or controlling behavior in the usual sense. It's a deeply ingrained pattern of thinking that equates their personal preferences with universal truths. And because they can't see this pattern in themselves, they can't understand why you seem so sensitive or defensive when they're "just trying to help."

Why your partner doesn't think anything is wrong

The biggest challenge in OCPD relationships is what psychologists call "ego-syntonic" symptoms (Hopwood et al., 2013). This fancy term means the behaviors feel natural and justified to the person exhibiting them. Unlike someone with depression who knows they feel terrible, or someone with anxiety who recognizes their fears as excessive, people with OCPD genuinely believe their rigid standards and controlling behaviors are reasonable responses to an inefficient, careless world.

Your partner looks around and sees chaos everywhere—dishes not loaded in the dishwasher with perfect efficiency, bills not filed in the optimal system, vacation plans that haven't been researched with appropriate thoroughness. From their perspective, someone needs to maintain standards around here, and unfortunately, that someone is always them.

This is completely different from Obsessive-Compulsive Disorder (OCD), which people often confuse with OCPD. Someone with OCD knows their compulsions are irrational. They wash their hands repeatedly while thinking, "This is crazy, but I can't stop." Someone with OCPD washes dishes in a very specific order while thinking, "This is obviously the most efficient method."

The key differences break down like this:

OCD involves unwanted intrusive thoughts and compulsions. The person recognizes these as problems and wants them to stop. They might think, "If I don't check the stove five times, something terrible will happen," while knowing logically that this doesn't make sense.

OCPD involves rigid preferences presented as logical necessities. The person sees their way as simply superior. They might say, "Obviously you need to check the stove twice before leaving the house—anything less is careless," and mean it completely.

People with OCD typically seek help because their symptoms interfere with their lives. People with OCPD resist help because they see their symptoms as solutions to other people's lack of care and attention to detail.

This creates a maddening dynamic for partners. You can't reason with someone who believes their position is perfectly reasonable. You can't compromise with someone who sees compromise as settling for inferior outcomes. And you can't get support from someone who thinks the real problem is your resistance to obviously better methods.

The four faces of OCPD in relationships

OCPD doesn't look the same in everyone. While all people with OCPD share certain core features—perfectionism, rigidity, need for control—these traits express themselves differently depending on the person's particular focus areas. Understanding your partner's specific subtype can help you make sense of their behavior patterns.

Controllers focus primarily on managing their environment and the people in it. These partners have detailed opinions about how household tasks should be completed, how money should be spent, how social events should be planned, and how problems should be solved. They frequently take over tasks you've started because you're "not doing it right." They may reorganize your belongings, critique your methods, or insist on approving decisions before you make them.

Lisa's husband Mark exemplifies this pattern. He has a specific way the dishwasher must be loaded ("geometric efficiency"), a preferred route for every destination ("I've timed all the alternatives"), and strong opinions about her clothing choices ("that color doesn't optimize your skin tone"). When Lisa tries to do things her own way, Mark either takes over or provides detailed correction instructions. He genuinely believes he's being helpful.

Workaholics channel their perfectionism into professional achievement and productivity. These partners struggle to relax, take minimal vacation time, and often work evenings and weekends. They may push you to be more ambitious or criticize what they see as laziness in others. Their identity is deeply tied to being productive and accomplished.

Jenny's wife Carol works 60-hour weeks and spends weekends on professional development courses. When Jenny suggests they take a spontaneous day trip, Carol responds with concern about "wasted time" that could be spent on more productive activities. Carol doesn't understand why Jenny seems unhappy with her dedication to success.

Moral Crusaders focus on ethical standards and doing things the "right" way. These partners have strong opinions about proper behavior, fairness, and social responsibility. They may criticize others' choices as selfish or careless and pride themselves on their integrity and moral consistency.

David's partner Tom insists on researching the ethical practices of every company they purchase from, spends considerable time writing complaint letters about poor service, and frequently points out when others are cutting in line, littering, or otherwise failing to follow social norms. Tom sees this as being a responsible citizen; David experiences it as exhausting moral surveillance.

List-Makers focus on organization, planning, and systematic approaches to life. These partners love detailed schedules, comprehensive lists, and thorough research before making decisions. They may become anxious or frustrated when plans change or when they feel unprepared for situations.

Rachel's husband Jake creates detailed itineraries for every trip, maintains multiple organizational systems for household management, and researches purchases exhaustively before buying anything. When Rachel suggests making spontaneous plans, Jake becomes visibly uncomfortable and immediately starts asking logistical questions that need to be resolved first.

Many people with OCPD show features of multiple subtypes, but usually one pattern dominates their relationship dynamic.

Self-assessment: Is your partner's behavior OCPD or something else?

Not every controlling or critical partner has OCPD. Sometimes relationship problems stem from stress, depression, anxiety, or simply incompatible personalities. Other times, what looks like OCPD might actually be narcissistic behavior or even emotional abuse.

Here's a assessment framework to help you determine if OCPD explains your relationship dynamic:

Perfectionism patterns: Does your partner have extremely high standards that seem unreasonable to others? Do they spend excessive time on tasks to get them "just right"? Are they genuinely distressed when things don't meet their standards, rather than just using perfectionism to control you?

Rigid thinking: Does your partner struggle to see alternative ways of doing things? When you suggest different approaches, do they respond with logical explanations about why their way is superior? Do they seem genuinely confused when others don't share their preferences?

Control vs. flexibility: Does your partner insist on doing things themselves because others won't do them correctly? Do they have trouble delegating or accepting help? When plans change unexpectedly, do they become anxious or frustrated rather than adapting easily?

Work and productivity focus: Is your partner a workaholic who struggles to relax? Do they have difficulty throwing things away because items might be useful someday? Are they more comfortable with tasks and projects than with emotional conversations?

Moral rigidity: Does your partner have strong opinions about right and wrong ways to behave? Do they criticize others for being careless, irresponsible, or inefficient? Do they see their standards as obviously correct rather than personal preferences?

The key distinguishing feature is **genuine belief in the superiority of their approach.** Someone with OCPD isn't trying to manipulate or control you for emotional satisfaction. They really believe their way is better and feel frustrated that you don't recognize this obvious truth.

This differs from:

Narcissistic behavior, where the person enjoys the power and control itself

Anxiety disorders, where perfectionism stems from fear rather than perceived superiority
Emotional abuse, where controlling behavior is designed to diminish your self-esteem

Stress responses, where perfectionism increases during difficult periods but decreases when stress resolves

Someone with OCPD will show these patterns consistently across multiple life areas and relationships, not just with you. They'll have similar conflicts with coworkers, family members, and friends who don't meet their standards.

The emotional cost of living with impossible standards

If you're living with someone who has OCPD, you're probably exhausted in ways that are hard to explain to others. Your partner isn't mean or deliberately cruel. They may be loving, responsible, and committed to the relationship. But their relentless standards and need for control create a particular kind of emotional drain.

You might find yourself:

Second-guessing your decisions before making them, trying to anticipate what your partner will think is wrong with your approach

Feeling incompetent in areas where you used to feel confident, because nothing you do seems to meet their standards

Walking on eggshells around household tasks, social plans, or daily decisions that should be simple and stress-free

Losing your sense of spontaneity because everything requires planning, research, or approval to avoid conflict

Feeling invisible as a person with valid preferences, since your partner's way is always presented as objectively better

Questioning your own judgment about what's reasonable or normal in relationships

This emotional toll is real and significant. Research shows that partners of people with personality disorders experience higher rates of depression, anxiety, and relationship dissatisfaction (Whisman & Baucom, 2012). You're not weak or oversensitive for struggling with this dynamic.

Why understanding OCPD changes everything

Learning about OCPD can be simultaneously validating and overwhelming. On one hand, finally having an explanation for your partner's behavior patterns provides tremendous relief. You're not imagining things, and you're not the problem.

On the other hand, personality disorders are deeply ingrained patterns that don't change easily. Your partner's rigid thinking and need for control aren't choices they're making—they're automatic responses that feel completely natural and justified.

But here's what understanding OCPD gives you:

Permission to stop taking it personally. When your partner criticizes your methods or takes over your tasks, it's not because you're incompetent. It's because they have a mental health condition that makes them unable to tolerate approaches different from their own.

A framework for responding differently. Instead of defending your choices or trying to prove your way is also valid, you can recognize that your partner's brain literally processes "different" as "wrong."

Realistic expectations for change. OCPD symptoms can improve with appropriate treatment, but expecting your partner to suddenly become flexible and easy-going isn't realistic. Change happens gradually and requires professional support.

Strategies for protecting your mental health. Knowing you're dealing with a personality disorder helps you establish appropriate boundaries and self-care practices.

Hope for improvement. While OCPD is challenging, many couples find ways to create more balanced, satisfying relationships when both partners understand what they're working with.

The goal isn't to diagnose your partner or use OCPD as an excuse for problematic behavior. The goal is to understand the underlying patterns so you can respond more effectively and protect your own well-being.

Moving forward with compassion and clarity

Your partner didn't choose to have OCPD, and their symptoms aren't intentionally designed to make your life difficult. They're operating from a genuine belief that their standards and methods are reasonable and helpful. This doesn't mean you have to accept behavior that harms your mental health, but it does mean you can stop trying to logic your way out of an illogical situation.

Someone with OCPD can't simply "relax their standards" or "be more flexible" any more than someone with diabetes can just "make more insulin." Their brain processes information in ways that make rigid thinking feel necessary and correct.

But understanding the condition also means recognizing that change is possible. With appropriate support, people with OCPD can learn to recognize their patterns, develop more flexibility, and create space for others' preferences and approaches.

Your job isn't to fix your partner or manage their symptoms. Your job is to understand what you're dealing with so you can make informed decisions about how to protect your own mental health while navigating this challenging relationship dynamic.

The following chapters will give you specific tools for communication, boundary-setting, self-care, and decision-making. But it all starts here, with the recognition that you're not crazy, you're not the problem, and your experiences make perfect sense given what you're dealing with.

You deserve to feel heard, valued, and respected in your relationship. OCPD might explain your partner's behavior, but it doesn't excuse treatment that leaves you feeling diminished or invisible.

The path forward requires both compassion for your partner's condition and fierce protection of your own well-being. Let's explore how to walk that path together.

Chapter 2: Inside the rigid mind

why your partner must control everything

Michael watched in familiar frustration as his wife Emma reorganized the dishwasher he'd just loaded. Again. She moved plates from one section to another, rearranged the silverware basket, and adjusted the angle of several bowls with the focused intensity of someone defusing a bomb.

"There," she said, closing the dishwasher door with satisfaction. "Now it'll clean properly."

Michael had loaded dishwashers successfully for fifteen years before marrying Emma. But somehow, his perfectly adequate loading method had become inadequate the moment he moved in with her. When he asked Emma why she needed to redo his work, she looked genuinely puzzled by the question.

"I just want it done right," she said, as if this explained everything.

And to Emma, it did explain everything. In her mind, there was a correct way to load a dishwasher that maximized cleaning efficiency and prevented damage to dishes. Michael's way wasn't wrong because she wanted to control him—it was wrong because it was objectively inferior to the optimal method. She was simply fixing a problem that needed fixing.

This is the heart of OCPD thinking: an absolute conviction that their way is not just better, but logically, obviously, practically superior. Understanding how this mindset develops and operates is crucial for anyone trying to navigate a relationship with someone who has this condition.

The perfectionism trap that never ends

Perfectionism in OCPD isn't the healthy drive for excellence that pushes athletes to train harder or students to study more carefully. It's a rigid, all-consuming need for things to be done exactly right, according to very specific internal standards that often seem arbitrary to others.

Your partner's perfectionism operates on several levels simultaneously:

Task perfectionism: Every activity has an optimal method that should be followed precisely. Loading dishwashers, folding laundry, planning trips, organizing files—all of these have correct procedures that shouldn't be compromised.

Outcome perfectionism: Results must meet extremely high standards. A "good enough" outcome feels unacceptable because it represents settling for mediocrity when excellence was achievable.

Process perfectionism: Not only must the end result be perfect, but the method used to achieve it must also be optimal. Taking shortcuts or using alternative approaches feels wrong even if they produce adequate results.

Timeline perfectionism: Tasks should be completed according to ideal schedules. Starting late, finishing early, or adjusting timelines based on circumstances feels chaotic and irresponsible.

What makes this particularly challenging for partners is that these perfectionist standards feel completely reasonable to the person with OCPD. They're not trying to make your life difficult—they genuinely cannot understand why you wouldn't want to do things the most effective way possible.

Research suggests that this perfectionism develops as a coping mechanism for underlying anxiety about chaos, failure, or loss of control (Egan et al., 2011). By maintaining extremely high standards and rigid procedures, people with OCPD create a sense of predictability and control in an unpredictable world.

But here's the trap: perfectionist standards are never truly achievable. There's always a way to do something better, faster, more efficiently, or more thoroughly. This creates a perpetual state of dissatisfaction where current efforts, no matter how good, never quite measure up to the ideal.

For your partner, this means constant vigilance. They can't relax and enjoy achievements because they're already focused on the next improvement that needs to be made. For you, it means your efforts are evaluated against impossible standards that leave little room for appreciation or satisfaction.

Fear drives the need for control

Beneath your partner's rigid standards and controlling behaviors lies a profound anxiety about what happens when things aren't done correctly. This isn't the specific phobia fear of something terrible happening if they don't check the stove five times (that's OCD). It's a more generalized dread of inefficiency, waste, mistakes, and the chaos that results from less-than-optimal choices.

People with OCPD often describe feeling physically uncomfortable when they observe inefficient methods or substandard results. Watching someone take a longer route to a destination, use an inferior organizational system, or make a decision without adequate research can create genuine distress.

This fear shows up in several ways:

Fear of waste: Using resources inefficiently feels morally wrong and practically harmful. This might mean spending hours researching the perfect purchase to save twenty dollars, or being unable to throw away items that might someday be useful.

Fear of inefficiency: Taking longer than necessary or using more steps than required feels intolerable. Your partner may take over tasks you're doing because they can complete them faster or better.

Fear of poor outcomes: Making decisions without thorough research and careful planning feels reckless. Your partner may resist spontaneous choices because they haven't had time to consider all possible alternatives and optimize the decision.

Fear of criticism: Being seen as careless, lazy, or irresponsible by others feels devastating. Your partner may insist on extremely high standards partly to avoid any possibility of being judged negatively.

Fear of lost opportunities: Not choosing the absolute best option means settling for something inferior when better was available. This can make simple decisions agonizing because of the pressure to identify the perfect choice.

These fears aren't irrational given your partner's worldview. If you believe there's always an optimal way to do things, then deviation from that optimal path really does represent unnecessary waste, inefficiency, and poor outcomes. The problem is that this worldview makes normal life extremely stressful and relationships very difficult.

Understanding that fear drives your partner's controlling behavior can help you respond with more compassion while still protecting your own needs. They're not trying to dominate you—they're trying to protect against outcomes that genuinely terrify them.

Why they see their behavior as justified

One of the most frustrating aspects of living with someone who has OCPD is their complete conviction that their standards and methods are reasonable. When you express frustration with their controlling behavior, they often respond with genuine confusion about why you're upset.

This happens because of what psychologists call "ego-syntonic" symptoms—behaviors that feel natural, logical, and justified to the person exhibiting them (Pinto et al., 2014). Your partner doesn't experience their rigidity as a problem that needs fixing. They experience it as a solution to problems that others create through carelessness and inefficiency.

From their perspective:

Their standards aren't unreasonably high—everyone else's are unreasonably low. When your partner insists on researching restaurants thoroughly before choosing one, they see this as responsible planning. Your preference for picking a place spontaneously feels reckless and likely to result in a disappointing meal.

Their methods aren't overly complicated—they're appropriately thorough. When your partner creates detailed systems for household organization, they see this as preventing chaos and saving time in the long run. Your more flexible approach feels disorganized and inefficient.

Their criticism isn't harsh—it's helpful feedback. When your partner points out better ways to do things, they genuinely believe they're providing useful information that will improve outcomes. Your defensive response feels ungrateful and illogical.

Their need for control isn't dominating—it's taking responsibility. When your partner takes over tasks or insists on specific approaches, they see this as ensuring quality results. Your resistance feels like you prefer inferior outcomes.

This creates an incredibly challenging dynamic for relationships. You can't reason with someone who believes their position is perfectly logical. You can't compromise with someone who sees compromise as accepting objectively worse outcomes. And you can't get empathy from someone who thinks your frustration is based on misunderstanding rather than legitimate concerns.

The key insight here is that your partner isn't being deliberately stubborn or controlling. They're operating from a fundamentally different set of assumptions about what's reasonable, necessary, and helpful in daily life.

The anxiety beneath the criticism

When your partner criticizes your methods or corrects your approach, it rarely feels like anxiety to you. It feels like judgment, control, or criticism. But understanding the emotional foundation beneath their behavior can help you respond more effectively.

Your partner's corrections and takeovers are often anxiety-management strategies. When they see something being done in a way that differs from their internal standard, it creates discomfort that feels urgent and necessary to address.

This anxiety manifests as:

Intrusive thoughts about better methods: Your partner can't stop thinking about more efficient ways to accomplish the task you're working on. These thoughts feel important and helpful rather than obsessive.

Physical discomfort with inefficiency: Watching suboptimal processes can create genuine physical tension, restlessness, or agitation that's relieved by taking corrective action.

Worry about negative consequences: Your partner may experience genuine concern that your approach will lead to poor results, wasted resources, or missed opportunities.

Responsibility anxiety: If they don't speak up about better methods, they feel complicit in accepting inferior outcomes when they could have helped improve things.

Understanding this anxiety doesn't mean you should accept constant criticism or correction. But it can help you recognize that your partner's behavior often stems from emotional discomfort rather than a desire to control or diminish you.

This realization can change how you respond to their criticism. Instead of defending your methods or arguing about whose approach is better, you might acknowledge their anxiety while maintaining your boundaries: "I can see you're worried about how I'm doing this. I appreciate your concern, and I'm comfortable with my approach."

Real couples navigating OCPD dynamics

Let's look at how three different couples have learned to understand and work with OCPD patterns in their relationships.

Sarah and James: The Project Management Challenge

Sarah has OCPD with strong Controller and List-Maker features. She approaches every household project with detailed planning, research, and systematic execution. When she and James decided to paint their living room, Sarah created a comprehensive project plan that included color research, paint quality comparisons, surface preparation schedules, and optimal weather timing.

James preferred a simpler approach: pick a color they both liked, buy paint, and spend a weekend painting. To Sarah, this felt reckless and likely to produce poor results. To James, Sarah's approach felt unnecessarily complicated and controlling.

Their breakthrough came when James started understanding Sarah's anxiety about waste and poor outcomes. He realized that her detailed planning wasn't about controlling him—it was about managing her fear of ending up with a color they'd regret or a paint job that would need redoing.

James learned to appreciate Sarah's research while maintaining some autonomy in the process. He'd review her findings and make collaborative decisions rather than dismissing her preparation as excessive. Sarah learned to present her research as information rather than directives, giving James space to participate in planning decisions.

The result wasn't perfect compromise—Sarah still does more planning than James would prefer, and James still makes faster decisions than Sarah finds comfortable. But they understand each other's perspectives and work together rather than against each other.

Maria and David: The Social Planning Struggle

David has OCPD with strong Moral Crusader tendencies. He believes social obligations should be handled responsibly, which means responding to invitations promptly, bringing appropriate gifts, and following proper etiquette. He feels genuinely anxious when Maria suggests showing up to parties without bringing anything or RSVPing at the last minute.

Maria is more spontaneous and relaxed about social conventions. She doesn't see the moral weight that David attaches to these behaviors and finds his elaborate preparation for simple social events exhausting.

Their pattern used to involve David becoming increasingly anxious about social obligations while Maria became increasingly resistant to what felt like arbitrary rules and excessive preparation. Arguments would escalate with David feeling like Maria was being irresponsible and Maria feeling like David was being controlling.

Their shift happened when Maria began recognizing David's genuine distress about social responsibilities. She realized that what felt like controlling behavior was actually anxiety about being seen as rude, careless, or disrespectful. David's elaborate preparation wasn't about impressing people—it was about meeting his internal standards for proper behavior.

Maria started offering to handle social obligations according to David's standards when his anxiety was high, while David learned to communicate his concerns as preferences rather than moral imperatives. They developed a system where David handles social planning for events that feel important to him, while Maria takes the lead on casual gatherings where his anxiety is lower.

Jennifer and Lisa: The Household Efficiency Conflict

Lisa has OCPD with strong Workaholic and Controller features. She approaches household management like a optimization project, developing systems for everything from meal planning to laundry scheduling. She genuinely enjoys creating efficient processes and feels satisfied when household tasks are completed according to optimal procedures.

Jennifer appreciates Lisa's organizational skills but feels overwhelmed by the constant pressure to follow specific systems for routine tasks. She doesn't share Lisa's satisfaction with optimization and finds the detailed procedures unnecessarily complicated.

Their conflict intensified when Jennifer started avoiding household tasks because she knew Lisa would critique or redo her efforts. Lisa became increasingly frustrated with having to handle everything herself while Jennifer felt increasingly incompetent and shut out of managing their shared home.

Their solution involved recognizing their fundamental differences in how they experience household management. Lisa finds optimization satisfying and energizing; Jennifer finds it stressful and draining. Instead of trying to make Jennifer appreciate Lisa's systems or trying to make Lisa relax her standards, they divided responsibilities according to their strengths.

Lisa handles tasks that benefit from systematic approaches—meal planning, budgeting, maintenance schedules. Jennifer handles tasks that require creativity and flexibility—decorating, entertaining, seasonal organizing. They created overlap areas where Lisa's systems provide structure but Jennifer has autonomy in execution.

The key in all these cases was shifting from trying to change each other to understanding each other. The OCPD partner learned to present their concerns as anxiety management rather than objective truth. The non-OCPD partner learned to recognize genuine distress beneath controlling behavior while maintaining appropriate boundaries.

Building understanding without losing yourself

Understanding your partner's OCPD doesn't mean accepting behavior that harms your mental health or diminishes your autonomy. Compassion and boundaries aren't mutually exclusive—in fact, healthy boundaries often make compassion easier to maintain.

Here's what understanding OCPD can and cannot do for your relationship:

What understanding provides:

- Context for behavior patterns that seem arbitrary or controlling
- Reduced tendency to take criticism and corrections personally
- Realistic expectations for change and improvement
- Strategies for responding to anxiety-driven behaviors
- Framework for collaborative problem-solving

What understanding doesn't provide:

- Excuse for behavior that damages your self-esteem or mental health
- Requirement to accept unreasonable demands or criticism
- Obligation to manage your partner's anxiety or accommodate all their preferences
- Solution to fundamental compatibility issues
- Guarantee that your relationship will improve

The goal is compassionate understanding that includes fierce protection of your own well-being. You can recognize that your partner's controlling behavior stems from anxiety while still insisting that they find ways to manage that anxiety that don't involve controlling you.

You can appreciate that their standards feel reasonable to them while maintaining your right to approach tasks differently. You can acknowledge their expertise in certain areas while preserving your autonomy in others.

Most importantly, you can understand that OCPD is a real condition that affects how your partner thinks and feels without using that understanding to justify accepting treatment that leaves you feeling diminished, criticized, or invisible.

The path forward requires both insight and action

OCPD creates predictable patterns in relationships, but those patterns aren't unchangeable. Understanding how your partner's mind works is the first step toward creating a more balanced dynamic, but it's only the first step.

The next stage involves learning specific strategies for communication, boundary-setting, and self-care that work with OCPD rather than against it. This means finding ways to honor your partner's need for order and control while preserving your own autonomy and well-being.

It also means helping your partner recognize how their anxiety-driven behaviors affect you, even when those behaviors feel completely justified to them. People with OCPD can learn to see their patterns and develop more flexible approaches, but this usually requires both professional support and patient, consistent feedback from partners.

Change happens gradually in OCPD relationships. Expecting sudden flexibility or relaxed standards isn't realistic. But expecting respectful treatment, collaborative decision-making, and space for your own preferences is completely reasonable.

Your partner's OCPD explains their behavior, but it doesn't excuse behavior that diminishes your sense of competence, autonomy, or value in the relationship. Understanding their condition is a tool for creating positive change, not a reason to accept an unsustainable dynamic.

The goal is a relationship where your partner's need for order coexists with your need for flexibility, where their expertise is valued without overwhelming your autonomy, and where both of your contributions are appreciated rather than one person's standards dominating all decisions.

This balance is achievable, but it requires both understanding and action. Understanding without boundaries leads to enabling. Boundaries without understanding lead to constant conflict. Together, they create the foundation for genuine improvement.

Key insights for moving forward:

Your partner's controlling behavior usually stems from anxiety about inefficiency, waste, or poor outcomes rather than desire to dominate you. This doesn't make the behavior acceptable, but it gives you better strategies for responding to it.

Their conviction that their way is superior isn't stubbornness—it's a core feature of how OCPD affects thinking. You can acknowledge their expertise while maintaining your right to different approaches.

Change happens when both partners understand what they're working with and develop strategies that honor each person's needs. This requires professional support, patience, and commitment from both people.

Understanding OCPD gives you permission to stop trying to logic your way out of an illogical situation and start building the skills you need to protect your well-being while navigating this challenging but potentially workable dynamic.

Chapter 3: The relationship impact nobody talks about

Karen sat in her car outside the grocery store, staring at her carefully organized shopping list. Three columns: items needed, preferred brands, and backup options if the preferred brands weren't available. Her husband Tom had spent twenty minutes the night before explaining why this system was more efficient than her usual approach of writing items down as she thought of them.

The list itself wasn't the problem. Tom's organizational system was actually quite useful. The problem was the familiar weight in her chest, the exhaustion that had nothing to do with the grocery shopping itself and everything to do with the constant feeling that her natural way of doing things was somehow inadequate.

Karen couldn't remember the last time she'd made a simple decision without anticipating Tom's analysis of why a different choice would have been better. She'd stopped suggesting restaurants because Tom would inevitably find reviews indicating superior options. She'd stopped buying gifts spontaneously because Tom preferred researching the optimal present for each recipient.

None of Tom's suggestions were unreasonable. His restaurant recommendations were usually excellent. His gift-giving research led to presents people genuinely appreciated. His grocery system did save time and reduce forgotten items.

But Karen felt like she was disappearing. Not because Tom was cruel or deliberately controlling, but because his constant optimization of her choices had eroded her confidence in her own judgment.

This is the hidden cost of OCPD relationships—the slow erosion of the non-OCPD partner's sense of competence, spontaneity, and autonomous decision-making. It happens gradually, with each small correction and improvement, until one day you realize you've stopped trusting your own instincts about basic life decisions.

The exhaustion that friends don't understand

Partners of people with OCPD experience a unique type of emotional fatigue that can be difficult to explain to others. Your friends might say, "At least your partner cares about doing things well," or "That sounds helpful—I wish my spouse was more organized." But they don't understand the cumulative impact of living with someone whose standards transform routine activities into performance evaluations.

This exhaustion has several components:

Decision fatigue from constant anticipation. Every choice you make requires mental energy to predict how your partner will respond, what improvements they'll suggest, and whether the resulting discussion will be worth it. Simple decisions become complex calculations about effort, conflict, and outcomes.

Emotional labor from managing their anxiety. You find yourself adjusting your behavior not because you agree with their preferences, but because you want to avoid the stress and disappointment they experience when things aren't done their way.

Cognitive overload from tracking their systems. Living with someone with OCPD often means learning and maintaining multiple organizational systems, procedures, and preferences that feel arbitrary but are important to your partner.

Performance anxiety in your own home. Tasks that should feel routine and comfortable become opportunities for evaluation and improvement. You lose the ability to relax into your natural rhythms and approaches.

Identity confusion from constant correction. When your partner regularly suggests better ways to do things, you begin to question your own competence and judgment. You may find yourself deferring to their expertise even in areas where you previously felt confident.

Research shows that partners of individuals with personality disorders experience significantly higher rates of depression, anxiety, and relationship distress compared to control groups (Clifton et al., 2007). The emotional toll is real and measurable, even when the relationship isn't abusive in traditional ways.

Many partners describe feeling like they're "walking on eggshells"— not because they fear explosive anger, but because they fear triggering their partner's distress about inefficiency or imperfection. This creates a hypervigilant state that's exhausting to maintain.

The slow erosion of spontaneity and confidence

One of the most significant impacts of OCPD relationships is the gradual loss of spontaneity and natural decision-making. Partners often report that they used to be more decisive, creative, and confident before adapting to their partner's need for optimization and control.

This happens through several mechanisms:

Analysis paralysis replacement. Your partner's tendency to research decisions thoroughly can gradually replace your intuitive decision-making process. You begin to feel irresponsible making choices without extensive analysis, even when the stakes are low.

Confidence erosion through comparison. Constant exposure to "better" ways of doing things can undermine your confidence in your own methods, even when your methods work perfectly well for your needs and preferences.

Spontaneity suppression. OCPD partners often struggle with unplanned activities because they haven't had time to research and optimize the experience. Over time, you may stop suggesting spontaneous activities to avoid their discomfort or lengthy planning discussions.

Creative constraint. The focus on optimal outcomes can crowd out experimentation, playfulness, and creative approaches that might not be efficient but could be enjoyable or meaningful.

Natural rhythm disruption. Everyone has personal rhythms for how they prefer to approach tasks, make decisions, and organize their time. Living with OCPD often means adapting to your partner's rhythms instead of finding a balance that works for both of you.

Jennifer describes this process: "I used to love cooking intuitively— tasting as I went, experimenting with ingredients, making it up as I went along. But my husband would watch and make suggestions about technique, timing, and ingredient ratios. His suggestions usually improved the dish, but I stopped enjoying the creative process. Now I follow recipes exactly and feel anxious when I want to deviate from instructions."

This isn't usually intentional on the OCPD partner's part. They're genuinely trying to be helpful by sharing their knowledge and improving outcomes. But the cumulative effect can be a significant loss of personal autonomy and creative expression for their partners.

Secondary mental health effects that compound over time

Living in an OCPD relationship creates stress that can trigger or worsen mental health conditions in the non-OCPD partner. These secondary effects often develop gradually and may not be immediately connected to the relationship dynamic.

Depression often emerges from the chronic feeling of inadequacy and loss of personal agency. When your natural approaches are constantly improved upon, it's easy to develop a sense of learned helplessness and loss of competence.

Anxiety can develop around decision-making, task completion, and anticipating your partner's responses. Many partners report developing generalized worry about "doing things wrong" that extends beyond their relationship.

Perfectionist tendencies may develop as a defense mechanism. If your partner's standards feel unavoidable, you might adopt perfectionist strategies to avoid criticism, even though perfectionism feels unnatural and stressful to you.

Social withdrawal often occurs when your partner's standards extend to social situations. You might decline invitations or avoid hosting events because the planning and execution requirements feel overwhelming.

Identity confusion can develop when your partner's expertise dominates so many life areas that you lose track of your own preferences, strengths, and decision-making abilities.

Resentment and anger may build over time, even though your partner's behavior isn't intentionally harmful. The accumulation of small corrections and improvements can create significant emotional buildup.

These secondary effects are particularly challenging because they're often invisible to others, including your partner. Your OCPD partner may genuinely believe they're being helpful and supportive, while you experience increasing distress and loss of self-confidence.

Impact on children that reverberates through generations

Children in OCPD households face unique challenges that can affect their development, self-esteem, and future relationships. The impact varies depending on the child's temperament, but certain patterns are common across these families.

Impossible standards become internalized expectations. Children may develop their own perfectionist tendencies as they try to meet the OCPD parent's standards or avoid their disappointment and anxiety when things aren't done correctly.

Natural childhood messiness becomes problematic. Age-appropriate exploration, experimentation, and learning through trial and error can trigger anxiety in the OCPD parent, leading to premature pressure for organization and precision.

Creativity and risk-taking are discouraged. The focus on optimal outcomes can inadvertently suppress children's willingness to try new things, make mistakes, or explore unconventional approaches.

Anxiety about parental approval increases. Children learn to anticipate the OCPD parent's standards and may become hypervigilant about potential criticism or correction.

Emotional expression becomes constrained. OCPD parents often struggle with emotional unpredictability and may inadvertently discourage emotional expression that feels chaotic or difficult to manage.

Independence development is delayed. The OCPD parent's need to ensure things are done correctly can interfere with children's natural progression toward autonomous decision-making and self-reliance.

Adult children from OCPD households often report:

- Difficulty making decisions without extensive research and analysis
- Perfectionist tendencies that feel compulsive rather than motivating
- Anxiety about being judged or criticized by authority figures
- Challenges with creative expression and spontaneous activities
- Hypervigilance about other people's standards and expectations

However, it's important to note that OCPD parents also provide significant benefits. They often create structured, predictable environments with high academic and behavioral standards. Many children from OCPD households develop strong work ethics, organizational skills, and achievement motivation.

The key is balance. Children need structure and standards, but they also need space for exploration, mistakes, and autonomous development. OCPD parents who recognize their condition can learn to provide guidance without overwhelming their children with impossible standards.

Financial and social consequences that extend beyond the couple

OCPD affects more than just the intimate relationship between partners. The condition often creates broader impacts on finances, social relationships, and extended family dynamics.

Financial impacts can be significant:

Over-researching purchases can lead to extensive time investments in finding optimal deals, sometimes spending hours to save modest amounts of money. While this can result in good purchases, the time cost may outweigh the financial benefits.

Difficulty with financial compromise occurs when the OCPD partner has strong opinions about optimal spending decisions. This can create conflict about purchases that the other partner considers reasonable but the OCPD partner sees as inferior choices.

Resistance to "unnecessary" spending on items that improve quality of life but don't meet objective criteria for value. This might include entertainment, convenience items, or experiences that feel wasteful to the OCPD partner.

Extensive research requirements for major purchases can delay important decisions while the OCPD partner gathers comprehensive information. This thoroughness can be beneficial but may also create frustration when urgent needs aren't met promptly.

Social impacts affect relationships beyond the couple:

Event planning anxiety can make social hosting stressful when the OCPD partner feels responsible for optimizing every detail of gatherings, from menu selection to guest list management.

Gift-giving pressure increases when the OCPD partner researches extensively to find the perfect present, potentially creating expectations that feel overwhelming to family and friends.

Social spontaneity decreases when the OCPD partner needs time to plan and research social activities, making it difficult to accept last-minute invitations or participate in unstructured gatherings.

Family relationship strain can develop when extended family members feel judged or criticized for their approaches to parenting, household management, or life choices.

Friendship maintenance becomes challenging when social activities require extensive planning or when the OCPD partner's standards create tension in group settings.

These broader impacts can create isolation for both partners. The non-OCPD partner may avoid social situations to prevent conflict, while the OCPD partner may feel misunderstood when others don't appreciate their efforts to optimize shared experiences.

The paradox of loving someone who improves everything

One of the most confusing aspects of OCPD relationships is that your partner's input often does improve outcomes. Their restaurant recommendations are usually excellent. Their travel planning creates smoother trips. Their organizational systems do save time and reduce stress.

This creates a challenging paradox: How do you address behavior that's simultaneously helpful and harmful? How do you express frustration with someone who's genuinely trying to make things better?

Many partners struggle with guilt about their negative feelings toward behavior that's intended to be supportive. They wonder if they're being ungrateful, lazy, or resistant to improvement. This internal conflict adds another layer of stress to an already challenging dynamic.

The key insight is that **impact matters more than intent.** Your partner's desire to help doesn't negate the negative impact their behavior has on your autonomy, confidence, and well-being. You can appreciate their expertise while still needing space for your own decision-making and approaches.

It's also important to recognize that improvement isn't always worth the cost. A restaurant meal that's 10% better isn't worth the stress of extensive research if you were happy with your original choice. An organizational system that saves fifteen minutes isn't worth adopting if it creates anxiety and feels unnatural.

You have the right to choose "good enough" over "optimal" in many life situations. Your partner's OCPD makes this choice feel illogical to them, but your mental health and autonomy are valid considerations that should influence household decisions.

When the relationship becomes a project to optimize

Perhaps the most challenging aspect of OCPD relationships is when your partner begins treating the relationship itself as a system that needs optimization. This might manifest as:

Relationship improvement research where your partner reads extensively about relationship strategies and tries to implement optimal approaches to communication, intimacy, and conflict resolution.

Performance tracking where your partner monitors relationship satisfaction, conflict frequency, or other metrics to identify areas for improvement.

Communication optimization where your partner develops systems for more efficient discussions, better conflict resolution, or improved emotional expression.

Activity planning where your partner researches and plans optimal approaches to shared activities, from date nights to vacation planning.

While some of this can be beneficial, it becomes problematic when the focus on optimization crowds out spontaneity, emotional authenticity, and natural relationship development. Relationships need space for imperfection, inefficiency, and organic growth.

When your partner treats the relationship as a project to be optimized, it can feel like you're being managed rather than loved. Your emotional responses may be seen as data points to be addressed rather than valid experiences to be understood.

This dynamic requires careful boundary-setting. You can appreciate your partner's investment in relationship improvement while maintaining your need for authentic emotional expression and natural relationship rhythms.

Recognizing that your experience is valid and predictable

If you recognize yourself in these descriptions, please understand that your experience is both valid and predictable. OCPD creates consistent patterns across relationships, and the challenges you're facing aren't unique to your specific situation or evidence of personal failure.

Many partners report feeling like they must be "too sensitive" or "resistant to improvement" when they struggle with their OCPD partner's behavior. This self-blame is understandable but misguided. You're responding normally to an abnormal amount of scrutiny, correction, and optimization pressure.

Your need for autonomy, spontaneity, and acceptance of "good enough" outcomes is completely reasonable. Your partner's OCPD makes these needs feel illogical to them, but that doesn't make your needs invalid.

The relationship challenges you're experiencing aren't evidence of incompatibility or relationship failure. They're predictable results of trying to balance one person's need for control and optimization with another person's need for autonomy and flexibility.

This understanding should provide both validation and hope. Validation that your struggles make complete sense given what you're dealing with. Hope that these patterns can be changed with appropriate understanding, strategies, and professional support.

Creating realistic expectations for improvement

Understanding OCPD's impact on relationships helps establish realistic expectations for change and improvement. Some aspects of your relationship dynamic can improve significantly with appropriate strategies and professional support. Others may require ongoing management rather than complete resolution.

What can improve:

- Your partner's awareness of how their behavior affects you
- Communication strategies that reduce defensiveness and conflict
- Boundary-setting that protects your autonomy while respecting their needs
- Division of responsibilities that leverages each person's strengths
- Your confidence and decision-making abilities
- Overall relationship satisfaction and emotional connection

What requires ongoing management:

- Your partner's basic need for order and control
- Their difficulty with spontaneous activities and decisions
- Their tendency to see their way as objectively superior

- Your need to maintain boundaries around their optimization attempts

- The balance between their expertise and your autonomy

The goal isn't to eliminate all OCPD-related challenges from your relationship. The goal is to create a dynamic where both people's needs are respected, where the OCPD partner's strengths are valued without overwhelming their partner's autonomy, and where both people feel heard and appreciated.

This balance is achievable, but it requires understanding, patience, and commitment from both partners. It also usually requires professional support to help both people develop new patterns and strategies.

Moving toward balance and mutual respect

The relationship impacts described in this chapter aren't inevitable or permanent. Many couples successfully navigate OCPD-related challenges and create satisfying, balanced relationships that honor both partners' needs.

The key is recognizing that these challenges are symptoms of a mental health condition rather than evidence of personal failure or fundamental incompatibility. This recognition opens the door to compassionate problem-solving rather than blame and defensiveness.

Your partner's OCPD explains their behavior but doesn't excuse behavior that significantly impacts your mental health and well-being. You can understand their need for control while maintaining your right to autonomy. You can appreciate their expertise while preserving your decision-making authority.

The path forward requires both accommodation and boundaries, both understanding and self-protection, both patience and insistence on respectful treatment. This balance is challenging to achieve but essential for long-term relationship health.

The following chapters will provide specific strategies for communication, boundary-setting, self-care, and decision-making that can help you create this balance while protecting your mental health and preserving the positive aspects of your relationship.

Remember: Your experiences are valid, your needs are reasonable, and your relationship challenges are treatable with appropriate understanding and support.

Chapter 4: Boundaries that actually work with rigid personalities

Rachel stood in her kitchen, watching her husband David reorganize the dishwasher for the third time this week. Each plate had to face the same direction. Each cup needed optimal water flow positioning. Each utensil required specific basket placement for maximum cleaning efficiency.

She'd tried everything. Asking nicely. Explaining that her loading method worked fine. Getting frustrated and walking away. Nothing stopped the inevitable reorganization that made her feel like a child who couldn't handle basic household tasks.

But last week, something shifted. Instead of defending her dishwasher loading or getting upset about his changes, Rachel tried a different approach.

"I can see you prefer a specific loading pattern," she said calmly. "I'm going to load it my way, and you're welcome to adjust it if you need to. But I won't be changing my approach."

David looked surprised. "But this way is more efficient—"

"I understand you think so," Rachel interrupted gently. "And you can certainly arrange it however makes you comfortable. I'm just letting you know that I'll continue loading it my way."

The conversation ended there. David did rearrange the dishwasher, but something felt different. Rachel hadn't defended, argued, or given up her approach. She'd simply stated her boundary and let David manage his own response to it.

This wasn't magic, and it didn't solve everything overnight. But it was the first time Rachel felt like she had any power in their household management dynamic. She'd discovered something crucial about boundaries with rigid personalities: **they work best when they're about your behavior, not your partner's.**

Why traditional boundary advice fails with OCPD

Most boundary advice assumes you're dealing with someone who can recognize and respect other people's limits. "Just tell them to stop." "Explain how their behavior affects you." "Set clear consequences for boundary violations."

These approaches often backfire with OCPD partners because they're based on a fundamental misunderstanding of how OCPD thinking works. Your partner doesn't see their suggestions, corrections, or takeovers as boundary violations. They see them as helpful improvements that any reasonable person would appreciate.

Traditional boundaries also assume that the other person is deliberately crossing lines for personal gain. OCPD boundaries are different because your partner genuinely believes their way is objectively better. They're not trying to control you for emotional satisfaction—they're trying to help you achieve superior outcomes.

This creates several challenges for conventional boundary-setting:

Explaining impact doesn't change behavior because your partner believes the long-term benefits of their improvements outweigh your temporary discomfort with their methods.

Asking them to stop feels unreasonable to them because you're essentially asking them to watch you do things inefficiently when they know better approaches.

Setting consequences can escalate conflict because your partner may see your boundaries as stubbornness or resistance to obviously beneficial feedback.

Compromise feels like settling for inferior outcomes when optimal solutions are available.

The solution isn't to abandon boundaries altogether. It's to design boundaries that work with OCPD thinking patterns rather than against them.

The "I Will/I Won't" boundary method specifically for OCPD

Effective OCPD boundaries focus on your choices and actions rather than trying to control your partner's responses. Instead of telling them what they can't do, you clearly state what you will and won't do. This approach respects their autonomy while protecting yours.

The framework looks like this:

"I will [your action/choice], and you're welcome to [their response option]."

This method works because it:

- Acknowledges their right to their preferences and responses

- Maintains your right to your own choices and approaches

- Removes the power struggle by not trying to change their behavior

- Reduces defensiveness by not criticizing their methods

- Creates clarity about what you're responsible for versus what they're responsible for

Here's how it sounds in practice:

Traditional boundary: "Stop reorganizing things after I clean them."
OCPD-effective boundary: "I will clean using my preferred methods, and you're welcome to adjust things afterward if you need to."

Traditional boundary: "Don't criticize my cooking while I'm making   dinner."

OCPD-effective boundary: "I will cook dinner my way, and you're welcome to share suggestions after I'm finished or cook it yourself next time."

Traditional boundary: "You can't take over every project I start." **OCPD-effective boundary:** "I will complete this project using my approach, and you can start your own version if you prefer different methods."

The key is that you're not trying to stop their behavior—you're protecting your right to your own behavior while allowing them to manage their response however they need to.

Let's look at how this works in different scenarios:

Household task boundaries:

- "I will do laundry on my schedule using my preferred method, and you're welcome to do additional loads if you need things done differently."

- "I will organize my workspace in a way that works for me, and you can arrange your areas however you prefer."

- "I will handle meal planning this week using my approach, and you can add to the grocery list or cook additional meals if you want other options."

Decision-making boundaries:

- "I will choose restaurants based on my criteria, and you're welcome to suggest alternatives or make your own reservations."

- "I will buy gifts based on my budget and preferences, and you can purchase additional items if you want to give something else."

- "I will plan our weekend activities, and you can research additional options or plan the following weekend your way."

Communication boundaries:

- "I will share my thoughts on this topic, and you're welcome to disagree or share your perspective."

- "I will make this decision with the information I have, and you can make different choices for situations you're handling."

- "I will express my feelings about this situation, and you can have whatever emotional response feels right to you."

Notice that none of these boundaries try to control your partner's response. You're simply claiming your right to your own choices while explicitly acknowledging their right to theirs.

Task and responsibility boundaries that end micromanagement

One of the most exhausting aspects of OCPD relationships is the constant micromanagement of routine tasks. Your partner doesn't just have opinions about how things should be done—they feel compelled to share improvements, take over incomplete tasks, or redo finished work to meet their standards.

Task boundaries work by clearly dividing responsibility so that each person has full autonomy over their designated areas. This reduces the overlap that creates opportunities for micromanagement while ensuring that both people's needs for competence and control are met.

Here's how to create effective task boundaries:

Complete ownership principle: Each person has full responsibility for specific tasks, including planning, execution, and evaluation. The other person can express preferences but cannot take over or redo completed work.

Expertise acknowledgment: Areas where one person has genuine expertise or strong preferences become their primary responsibility, with input from the other person welcome but not required.

Rotation agreements: Tasks that both people care about can rotate on agreed schedules, with each person having complete control during their designated periods.

Backup systems: Clear procedures for what happens when the responsible person is unavailable, sick, or overwhelmed, preventing default takeover by the OCPD partner.

Quality standards discussion: Explicit conversations about minimum acceptable standards versus optimal outcomes, with agreements about when "good enough" is genuinely acceptable.

Practical examples of task boundary division:

Household management:

- Person A handles all grocery shopping, meal planning, and cooking, with Person B responsible for cleanup and kitchen organization

- Person B manages all household repairs, maintenance scheduling, and service provider communication, with Person A handling decor and organization decisions

- Each person manages their own laundry completely, with shared items handled on alternating weeks

Financial management:

- Person A handles day-to-day spending decisions up to agreed limits, with Person B managing investment research and long-term planning

- Each person has complete autonomy over their personal spending allocation, with joint decisions required only for major purchases

- One person handles bill paying and account management, with monthly reviews instead of ongoing involvement from both partners

Social planning:

- Person A plans all social activities for the first half of each month, with Person B responsible for the second half

- Each person handles relationships with their own family completely, including gift-giving, event attendance, and communication

- Work-related social obligations are managed by the person whose job is involved, with input from the partner welcome but not required

The key to making task boundaries work is **genuine handoff of control.** The OCPD partner must agree to accept the other person's methods and outcomes in their designated areas, even when they see opportunities for improvement. The non-OCPD partner must agree to handle their responsibilities without expecting the OCPD partner to lower their standards in areas they control.

This isn't about creating rigid separation—it's about reducing the constant negotiation and takeover that exhausts both partners.

Emotional boundaries that protect your mental health

OCPD partners often struggle to understand how their helpful suggestions and corrections affect their partner's emotional well-being. They see their feedback as useful information rather than criticism, so they may continue offering improvements even when their partner feels overwhelmed or demoralized.

Emotional boundaries protect your psychological space while allowing your partner to maintain their natural tendency to optimize and improve. These boundaries focus on managing your emotional exposure rather than changing your partner's communication style.

Information boundaries control how much input you receive about your methods and choices:

- "I will ask for your opinion when I want feedback about my approach. Otherwise, I prefer to handle this myself."

- "I appreciate that you have ideas about better methods. I'll consider them after I finish what I'm working on."

- "I can see you have thoughts about how I'm doing this. I'm going to complete it my way first, and then I'm happy to hear your suggestions."

Timing boundaries create space for you to process and respond rather than feeling pressured to immediately incorporate their suggestions:

- "I hear that you have ideas for improving this. Let me finish what I'm doing, and then we can discuss alternatives."

- "I appreciate your research on this topic. I need some time to consider your findings before making any changes."

- "I understand you've found a better approach. I'm going to try my method first, and we can compare results."

Emotional safety boundaries protect you from taking on responsibility for your partner's anxiety about suboptimal outcomes:

- "I can see you're concerned about my approach. I'm comfortable with my choice, and I hope you can find a way to be okay with it too."

- "I understand this method makes you anxious. I'm confident in my ability to handle any problems that come up."

- "I know you prefer a different approach. I'm willing to accept the consequences of my choice."

Competence boundaries protect your sense of capability and decision-making authority:

- "I appreciate your expertise in this area. I'm choosing to handle this situation based on my own judgment."

- "I understand you have more experience with this. I'm still going to approach it my way so I can learn from the experience."

- "I can see why your method would work well. I prefer to use my approach for this particular situation."

These boundaries require practice because they feel foreign at first. You're not used to claiming authority over your own choices when your partner has strong opinions about better alternatives. But emotional boundaries aren't about being stubborn or rejecting good advice—they're about maintaining your autonomy and mental health while living with someone whose brain is wired to see improvement opportunities everywhere.

The Broken Record technique for boundary enforcement

The Broken Record technique is particularly effective with OCPD partners because it avoids the detailed discussions and justifications that can trigger their problem-solving instincts. Instead of getting pulled into debates about whose method is better, you calmly repeat your boundary statement until the conversation ends.

Here's how it works:

Choose a simple, clear boundary statement that you can repeat exactly. Avoid explaining, justifying, or elaborating on your reasons.

Repeat the statement calmly each time your partner tries to discuss, debate, or change your boundary. Don't vary the wording or add new information.

Stay emotionally neutral. Don't get defensive, frustrated, or drawn into explaining why their alternative isn't what you want.

End the conversation when it becomes circular. You can simply say, "I think we've covered this topic completely" and change the subject or leave the room.

Here's what it looks like in practice:

Partner: "But if you organize it this way, it'll be much more efficient." **You:** "I'm going to organize it my way." **Partner:** "I just think you'd save time if you tried this method." **You:** "I'm going to organize it my way." **Partner:** "Can you at least look at this article about better organization systems?" **You:** "I'm going to organize it my way." **Partner:** "I don't understand why you won't consider a better approach." **You:** "I'm going to organize it my way. I think we've covered this topic completely."

The technique works because:

It doesn't provide new information for your partner's problem-solving brain to process and counter-argue.

It avoids defending your choice, which would invite detailed discussion about the merits of different approaches.

It stays focused on your decision rather than getting pulled into evaluating your partner's alternative.

It ends the conversation before it can escalate into frustration or conflict.

It demonstrates consistency in your boundary without being aggressive or dismissive.

The Broken Record technique can feel uncomfortable at first, especially if you're used to explaining your choices or trying to help your partner understand your perspective. But with OCPD partners, detailed explanations often trigger more suggestions and problem-solving rather than acceptance of your boundary.

Personal Boundary Mapping Exercise

Understanding your current boundaries and identifying areas that need strengthening requires honest assessment of where you feel respected versus where you feel overwhelmed or controlled. This exercise helps you create a clear picture of your boundary needs.

Step 1: Current Boundary Assessment

For each life area, rate your current sense of autonomy on a scale from 1 (completely controlled by partner) to 10 (complete personal autonomy):

Household tasks (cleaning, organizing, maintenance)

- Current autonomy level: ___
- Areas where you feel micromanaged: ___
- Tasks you avoid because of partner's standards: ___

Decision-making (purchases, plans, choices)

- Current autonomy level: ___
- Decisions your partner frequently questions or improves: ___
- Choices you run by your partner to avoid conflict: ___

Personal time (hobbies, relaxation, social activities)

- Current autonomy level: ___
- Activities your partner has opinions about: ___
- Time you spend managing their standards instead of enjoying yourself: ___

Communication (expressing opinions, sharing feelings, making requests)

- Current autonomy level: ___
- Topics where you edit yourself to avoid their corrections: ___
- Feelings you don't share because they'll be analyzed or improved: ___

Step 2: Priority Boundary Areas

Identify the three areas where boundary improvements would have the biggest positive impact on your well-being:

1. Priority area: ___ Why this matters: ___ Current challenge: ___

2. Priority area: ___ Why this matters: ___ Current challenge: ___

3. Priority area: ___ Why this matters: ___ Current challenge: ___

Step 3: Specific Boundary Statements

For each priority area, write specific "I will/I won't" boundary statements:

Priority Area 1:

- I will: ___
- I won't: ___
- My partner is welcome to: ___

Priority Area 2:

- I will: ___
- I won't: ___
- My partner is welcome to: ___

Priority Area 3:

- I will: ___
- I won't: ___
- My partner is welcome to: ___

Step 4: Implementation Planning

For each boundary, identify:

When you'll communicate this boundary: ___ **What resistance you expect:** ___ **How you'll use Broken Record technique:** ___ **What support you need:** ___

Step 5: Success Indicators

How will you know your boundaries are working?

What you'll feel more of: (confidence, energy, autonomy) **What you'll feel less of:** (anxiety, resentment, exhaustion) **Specific behavioral changes you'll notice:** ___

This mapping exercise isn't a one-time activity. Boundaries need regular assessment and adjustment as your relationship dynamics change and your confidence grows.

Managing the initial resistance and adjustment period

Setting boundaries with an OCPD partner often creates an initial period of confusion, frustration, and testing. Your partner is used to having input into your choices, and they may interpret your new boundaries as rejection of their help or evidence that you don't value their expertise.

Here's what to expect and how to manage this transition:

Increased suggestions and corrections as your partner tries to understand why you're suddenly resistant to obviously helpful feedback. They may double down on their efforts to demonstrate the benefits of their approaches.

Emotional responses including hurt feelings that you don't want their help, frustration that you're choosing inferior methods, or anxiety about the suboptimal outcomes they fear will result.

Testing behaviors where your partner pushes against your boundaries to see if you really mean them or if they can find exceptions and special circumstances.

Temporary relationship tension as both of you adjust to a new dynamic where your partner has less influence over your choices and methods.

Your own discomfort as you practice claiming authority over your decisions and resist the urge to explain or justify your boundaries.

Strategies for managing this adjustment period:

Stay consistent with your boundary statements even when your partner seems hurt or frustrated by them. Inconsistency teaches them that enough pressure will get you to abandon your limits.

Acknowledge their feelings without changing your boundaries. "I can see you're concerned about my approach. I understand this is frustrating for you, and I'm still going to handle it my way."

Avoid JADE (Justify, Argue, Defend, Explain). The more you explain your boundaries, the more material you give your partner's problem-solving brain to work with in trying to change your mind.

Focus on appreciation for the areas where your partner does respect your boundaries, even if they're still struggling with others.

Take care of yourself during this transition. Setting boundaries is emotionally taxing, especially when you're not used to claiming authority over your own choices.

Seek support from friends, family, or a therapist who understand what you're working on and can encourage you when the process feels difficult.

Most importantly, expect that this adjustment will take time. Your partner has spent years believing that their input improves your choices. Learning to respect your autonomy even when they see better alternatives requires significant mental and emotional adjustment.

Building collaborative decision-making within boundary framework

Effective boundaries with OCPD partners don't eliminate collaboration—they create space for healthier collaboration based on mutual respect rather than one person's standards dominating all decisions.

Once your basic boundaries are established, you can begin inviting your partner's input in ways that preserve your autonomy while benefiting from their expertise.

Selective consultation: "I'm planning our vacation, and I'd love your research help on hotels once I narrow down the destination."

Expertise utilization: "You're really good at finding the best deals. Could you help me research options for this purchase I'm planning to make?"

Collaborative timing: "I want to try my approach first, and then I'd appreciate hearing your thoughts on what worked and what could be improved."

Optional input: "I'm working on this project. If you have suggestions, I'm happy to hear them, but I may or may not incorporate them depending on my goals."

Structured feedback: "I'd like your opinion on this decision. Can you give me your top two suggestions without going into detailed analysis of all the alternatives?"

This approach allows you to benefit from your partner's analytical skills and expertise while maintaining control over how much input you receive and how you use it.

The key is that collaboration becomes a choice you make rather than something that automatically happens because your partner has strong opinions about optimal approaches.

Creating sustainable boundary practices

Boundaries aren't a one-time conversation—they're an ongoing practice that requires maintenance and adjustment. With OCPD partners, this is especially true because their brain continues to identify improvement opportunities, and you continue to need space for your own approaches and decisions.

Regular boundary check-ins help you assess what's working and what needs adjustment. Monthly conversations about how the boundary agreements are functioning can prevent small issues from becoming major conflicts.

Boundary refinement happens as you gain confidence and clarity about your needs. You might start with basic boundaries about household tasks and gradually extend them to financial decisions, social planning, or parenting approaches.

Appreciation practices help both partners recognize the benefits of the boundary system. Your partner may begin to appreciate having less responsibility for managing all household decisions, while you benefit from reduced criticism and increased autonomy.

Flexibility within structure allows for special circumstances while maintaining your basic boundary framework. You might accept more input during stressful periods while returning to your normal boundaries when things stabilize.

Professional support can be invaluable for both partners as you navigate this process. A therapist who understands OCPD can help your partner develop tolerance for your different approaches while helping you maintain appropriate boundaries.

The goal isn't to eliminate all areas of overlap and collaboration. It's to create a relationship dynamic where both people feel respected, where your partner's strengths are valued without overwhelming your autonomy, and where conflicts about methods and standards don't dominate your interactions.

Boundaries with OCPD partners require patience, consistency, and self-compassion. You're learning to claim authority over your own life while living with someone whose brain is wired to see improvement opportunities everywhere. This balance is challenging but absolutely achievable with the right approach and support.

Your boundaries aren't mean, selfish, or resistant to improvement. They're necessary protection for your mental health and autonomy in a relationship with someone who genuinely believes their way is superior. You deserve space to make your own choices, use your own methods, and learn from your own experiences, even when your partner can see more efficient alternatives.

Clear scripts and strategies for setting limits without triggering explosive reactions

The boundary techniques in this chapter work because they respect your partner's OCPD thinking patterns while protecting your own needs. They acknowledge your partner's expertise and preferences without requiring you to subordinate your autonomy to their standards.

These boundaries reduce explosive reactions because they don't attack your partner's competence or suggest their methods are wrong. Instead, they create parallel paths where both people can approach tasks and decisions according to their own preferences.

This isn't about winning or proving whose approach is better. It's about creating sustainable relationship dynamics where both people feel respected and valued, where your partner's need for control coexists with your need for autonomy, and where conflicts about methods don't overwhelm your connection and appreciation for each other.

Chapter 5: Communication strategies for the criticism minefield

Alex dreaded the moment his wife Carmen would walk into the kitchen while he was cooking. Not because she was mean or hostile, but because the helpful suggestions were endless and somehow always made him feel incompetent.

"If you cut the onions smaller, they'll cook more evenly," she'd say, watching over his shoulder.

"The pan should be hotter before you add the oil—you'll get better searing that way."

"Did you know that adding salt earlier in the process helps draw out more flavor?"

Each suggestion was technically accurate. Carmen had taken several cooking classes and genuinely knew more about culinary techniques than Alex did. But by the time dinner was ready, Alex felt like he'd failed a performance evaluation rather than prepared a meal for his family.

Last Tuesday, Alex tried something different. When Carmen started her usual suggestions, instead of getting defensive or trying to explain his methods, he said, "You're absolutely right that smaller onions cook more evenly, and I like the rustic look of bigger pieces for this particular dish. Both approaches work well."

Carmen paused, looking slightly confused. She'd expected either acceptance of her suggestion or an argument about cooking methods.

Alex's response acknowledged her expertise while maintaining his choice—something she hadn't encountered before.

"I guess both ways can work," she said slowly.

"Exactly," Alex replied. "Your way optimizes even cooking, and my way optimizes the visual presentation I'm going for tonight."

For the first time in months, Carmen watched him cook without offering additional corrections. She'd received the acknowledgment her expertise deserved, while Alex had maintained his autonomy without triggering her need to prove her methods were superior.

This interaction illustrates a crucial insight about communicating with OCPD partners: **they don't need you to adopt their methods, but they do need you to acknowledge that their methods have merit.**

The "Both/And" approach to rigid thinking

OCPD thinking operates in either/or patterns. Either there's a right way to do something, or there's a wrong way. Either you're being efficient, or you're being wasteful. Either you're doing it correctly, or you're making mistakes that need correction.

This binary thinking creates endless conflicts because most life situations actually have multiple valid approaches. Your way of loading the dishwasher works fine. Your partner's way also works fine. But OCPD thinking struggles to hold both truths simultaneously.

The "Both/And" approach helps your partner's brain make space for multiple valid approaches by explicitly acknowledging that their method has benefits while maintaining that your method also has benefits. Instead of getting trapped in debates about which approach is superior, you create a framework where both approaches can coexist.

Here's how it works:

Instead of: "My way works just fine." **Try:** "Your way maximizes efficiency, and my way works well for my priorities."

Instead of: "I don't need to do it your way." **Try:** "I can see how your method would save time, and I prefer my approach for this situation."

Instead of: "Stop telling me how to do everything." **Try:** "I appreciate that you know several effective methods. I'm choosing to use this approach today."

The key elements of effective "Both/And" communication:

Acknowledge the benefits of your partner's approach first. This addresses their need to have their expertise recognized and reduces their urgency to prove their method is superior.

Use connecting words like "and," "also," and "both" instead of "but," "however," and "instead." These words create inclusion rather than opposition.

Be specific about why you're choosing your approach without criticizing theirs. Focus on your preferences, priorities, or circumstances rather than suggesting their method is wrong.

Maintain confident energy about your choice. Uncertainty in your voice suggests you're not really convinced your way is valid, which invites more persuasion from your partner.

End the comparison cleanly without leaving space for debate about which approach is objectively better.

Let's look at how this sounds across different scenarios:

Household task conflicts:

- "You're right that folding towels that way saves space, and I like the way they look when I fold them my way."

- "I can see how your cleaning order is more efficient, and I prefer to start with the areas that bother me most."

- "That's definitely a thorough way to organize the garage, and I'm planning to use a simpler system that works for how I think about these items."

Financial decisions:

- "You've found some great research on the best value options, and I've decided to prioritize convenience over savings for this purchase."

- "I appreciate how much time you spent comparing prices, and I'm comfortable with this choice based on my budget priorities."

- "You're absolutely right that waiting for a sale would save money, and I'd rather buy it now for the immediate benefit."

Social planning:

- "I can see why planning ahead would reduce stress, and I'm excited about being spontaneous for this particular event."

- "You've identified some really interesting options through your research, and I'm drawn to this choice based on what sounds fun to me right now."

- "That venue would definitely provide the most value, and I prefer this location for the atmosphere it offers."

Parenting decisions:

- "You're right that this approach has proven benefits, and I want to try this alternative method based on what I know about our child's personality."

- "I can see the logic in that strategy, and I think this approach fits better with our family's current needs."

- "That's definitely a thorough way to handle this situation, and I prefer a more flexible approach for this particular issue."

The "Both/And" framework works because it satisfies your partner's need to have their expertise acknowledged while preserving your autonomy to make different choices. Your partner's OCPD brain can relax because their superior method has been recognized, even though you're not adopting it.

Scripts for common OCPD conflicts

Certain conflicts appear in almost every OCPD relationship. Having prepared responses for these recurring situations reduces the emotional energy you spend navigating criticism and corrections while helping your partner feel heard and respected.

Scenario 1: Task takeover *Your partner starts redoing or taking over something you're working on*

OCPD partner says: "Here, let me finish this—it'll be faster if I do it." **Your response options:**

- "I can see you know a quicker method, and I'm enjoying doing it my way right now."

- "You're definitely faster at this than I am, and I want to complete it myself this time."

- "I appreciate the offer to help, and I'd prefer to finish what I started."

Scenario 2: Method criticism *Your partner points out more efficient or better ways to do what you're doing*

OCPD partner says: "If you do it this way instead, you'll get much better results." **Your response options:**

- "You're probably right that would improve the outcome, and I'm satisfied with the results I'm getting this way."

- "I can see how that method would be more effective, and I prefer my approach for this situation."

- "That's good information to have. I'm planning to stick with this method today."

Scenario 3: Decision questioning *Your partner suggests you haven't researched or considered enough factors before making a choice*

OCPD partner says: "Don't you think you should research this more thoroughly before deciding?" **Your response options:**

- "You're right that more research might reveal better options, and I'm comfortable making this decision with the information I have."

- "I appreciate how thoroughly you research decisions, and I'm choosing to prioritize speed over optimization for this choice."

- "That's definitely one approach to decision-making, and I'm confident in this choice based on my priorities."

Scenario 4: Standards criticism *Your partner expresses concern that your standards aren't high enough*

OCPD partner says: "This isn't really up to the standard we usually maintain." **Your response options:**

- "You're right that we could do this to a higher standard, and I think this level works well for this particular situation."

- "I can see that this doesn't meet your usual standards, and I'm satisfied with this outcome."

- "You definitely have higher standards than I do for this, and I'm comfortable with this result."

Scenario 5: Efficiency concerns *Your partner worries you're wasting time, money, or resources*

OCPD partner says: "There's a much more efficient way to handle this." **Your response options:**

- "You're absolutely right that your way would be more efficient, and I value other factors more than efficiency for this task."

- "I can see how that approach would save time, and I prefer my method for reasons that matter to me."

- "That's definitely a more streamlined approach, and I'm choosing to prioritize enjoyment over efficiency right now."

Scenario 6: Planning pressure *Your partner wants more detailed planning than you think is necessary*

OCPD partner says: "We really should plan this out more carefully to avoid problems." **Your response options:**

- "You're right that more planning would prevent potential issues, and I'm comfortable handling problems as they come up."

- "I can see how thorough planning reduces stress for you, and I actually enjoy figuring things out spontaneously."

- "That level of planning would definitely improve our chances of success, and I prefer a more flexible approach."

Notice that each response follows the "Both/And" pattern: acknowledging the validity of your partner's perspective while maintaining your different choice. This reduces the likelihood that your partner will escalate their persuasion efforts because they've received the recognition their expertise deserves.

De-escalation techniques for perfectionist rage

OCPD partners sometimes experience intense frustration when they encounter inefficiency, poor outcomes, or resistance to obviously superior methods. This isn't the same as narcissistic rage (which is about control and dominance) or borderline rage (which is about fear of abandonment). Perfectionist rage stems from genuine distress about suboptimal outcomes and waste of resources.

Understanding the source of this frustration helps you respond in ways that address the underlying anxiety rather than escalating the conflict.

Validation without agreement acknowledges your partner's distress without accepting that their standards should govern the situation:

- "I can see you're really frustrated by this approach."

- "It's clearly distressing to you when things aren't done optimally."

- "I understand this situation creates anxiety for you."

Anxiety acknowledgment recognizes the fear beneath the frustration:

- "I can see you're worried about the outcome when things aren't done your preferred way."

- "I understand you feel responsible for preventing problems that you can see coming."

- "It sounds like you're concerned about waste/inefficiency/poor results."

Responsibility clarification helps your partner understand that you're taking responsibility for your choices and any consequences:

- "I understand you're concerned about how this will turn out. I'm prepared to handle any problems that arise."

- "I can see you think this approach might cause issues. I'm willing to accept those consequences."

- "I hear that you're worried about the results. I'm comfortable with the risk I'm taking."

Emotional space offering gives your partner permission to have their feelings without requiring you to change your approach:

- "I can see this is really bothering you. Would it help to talk about what specifically worries you?"

- "I understand this creates stress for you. How can I support you while still handling this my way?"

- "I can tell this is frustrating. What would help you feel better about the situation?"

Redirection to their control areas reminds your partner of the many things they do control and can optimize:

- "I know this isn't how you'd handle it. You can definitely approach it your way when you're in charge of similar situations."

- "I appreciate that you see better methods. You're welcome to use those approaches for tasks you're managing."

- "I understand you prefer different strategies. You have complete freedom to optimize the things you're responsible for."

When perfectionist rage escalates:

Stay calm and lower your voice rather than matching their intensity. Escalation feeds more escalation.

Avoid detailed discussions about methods, benefits, or outcomes during emotional peaks. Save problem-solving conversations for when both people are calm.

Set temporary boundaries if needed: "I can see you're very upset about this. Let's continue this conversation when we're both feeling calmer."

Don't take responsibility for managing their emotions: "I understand you're frustrated. I trust you to find ways to cope with that frustration."

Maintain your boundaries even when they're emotional: "I can see how much this bothers you, and I'm still going to handle it my way."

The goal isn't to eliminate your partner's frustration about suboptimal outcomes—that's part of how their brain works. The goal is to respond to their emotion without abandoning your autonomy or getting pulled into proving whose approach is better.

Using their values to motivate change

OCPD partners are more likely to modify their behavior when the change aligns with their existing values of efficiency, responsibility, and optimization. Instead of asking them to relax their standards or be more flexible (which feels like lowering their performance), you can frame relationship improvements in ways that appeal to their natural motivations.

Efficiency framing presents relationship changes as ways to reduce wasted time and energy:

- "I've noticed that when we spend twenty minutes discussing the best way to load the dishwasher, we could have loaded it twice in that time. What if we each just loaded it our own way?"

- "It seems like we both spend a lot of energy on these method discussions. Would it be more efficient to divide up responsibilities so each person can optimize their own areas?"

- "I'm wondering if there's a more streamlined way to make household decisions that doesn't require us to research every option together."

Relationship optimization frames changes as improvements to relationship performance:

- "I've been thinking about how to optimize our communication so we spend less time in conflict and more time enjoying each other."

- "What if we could design a system where both of us feel appreciated for our contributions instead of defensive about our methods?"

- "I'm interested in finding approaches that let us both use our strengths without stepping on each other's areas."

Goal achievement focuses on desired outcomes rather than process changes:

- "Our goal is having a peaceful household where both of us feel competent. What systems would help us achieve that?"

- "We both want to make good decisions efficiently. How can we structure our decision-making to accomplish that?"

- "The end result we both want is feeling appreciated and valued. What would need to change for both of us to feel that way?"

Problem-solving collaboration invites your partner to apply their analytical skills to relationship challenges:

- "I've identified a problem in how we handle household tasks, and I'd love your help brainstorming solutions."

- "There seems to be an inefficiency in our communication patterns. Would you be interested in researching better approaches?"

- "I think there might be a systematic way to reduce the frustration we both feel about these recurring conflicts."

Performance improvement appeals to their desire to excel in all areas:

- "I'm wondering how we can both perform at our best in this relationship instead of feeling like we're working against each other."

- "What would it look like if we were both operating at peak efficiency in our partnership?"

- "How can we optimize our relationship so both of us feel successful and appreciated?"

This approach works because you're not asking your partner to abandon their values—you're asking them to apply those values to relationship improvement. Their analytical skills and drive for optimization become assets for creating better relationship dynamics rather than obstacles to overcome.

Communication template library for ten scenarios

Having prepared responses for common OCPD relationship conflicts reduces the emotional energy you spend navigating these situations while increasing the likelihood of productive outcomes.

Template 1: Unsolicited advice *Situation: Your partner offers suggestions when you haven't asked for input*

Initial response: "I can see you have ideas about this. I'm going to handle it my way right now."

If they persist: "I appreciate that you want to help. I'm not looking for suggestions at the moment."

If they continue: "I understand you see better methods. I'm choosing my approach for this situation."

Template 2: Task criticism *Situation: Your partner points out flaws or inefficiencies in your work*

Initial response: "You're right that could be improved, and I'm satisfied with this result."

If they persist: "I can see you notice areas for optimization. I'm comfortable with my outcome."

If they continue: "I understand this doesn't meet your standards, and it works for my needs."

Template 3: Method takeover *Situation: Your partner starts doing something you're working on*

Initial response: "I can see you know a faster way. I want to complete this myself."

If they persist: "I appreciate that you're trying to help. I prefer to finish what I started."

If they continue: "I understand you can do this more efficiently. I'm enjoying doing it my own way."

Template 4: Decision questioning *Situation: Your partner suggests your choice isn't well-researched*

Initial response: "You're right that more research might reveal better options, and I'm comfortable with my decision."

If they persist: "I can see you prefer more thorough analysis. I'm confident in this choice."

If they continue: "I understand you'd want more information. I'm satisfied with what I know."

Template 5: Standards pressure *Situation: Your partner indicates your standards aren't high enough*

Initial response: "You definitely maintain higher standards than I do for this, and I'm comfortable with this level."

If they persist: "I can see this doesn't meet your usual quality expectations. This works for me."

If they continue: "I understand you'd do this more thoroughly. I'm satisfied with this approach."

Template 6: Efficiency concerns *Situation: Your partner worries you're being wasteful or inefficient*

Initial response: "You're absolutely right that would be more efficient, and I'm prioritizing other factors."

If they persist: "I can see how that approach would optimize results. I prefer my method for this situation."

If they continue: "I understand efficiency is important to you. I'm balancing different priorities."

Template 7: Planning pressure *Situation: Your partner wants more detailed preparation than you think necessary*

Initial response: "You're right that more planning would prevent problems, and I'm comfortable handling issues as they arise."

If they persist: "I can see how thorough planning reduces your stress. I prefer more spontaneous approaches."

If they continue: "I understand you like comprehensive preparation. I'm choosing flexibility for this situation."

Template 8: Perfectionist frustration *Situation: Your partner becomes upset about suboptimal outcomes*

Initial response: "I can see you're frustrated by this approach. I'm willing to accept the results."

If they escalate: "I understand this creates anxiety for you. I'm prepared to handle any consequences."

If they continue: "I can tell this really bothers you. I'm comfortable with the risk I'm taking."

Template 9: Control attempts *Situation: Your partner tries to manage your schedule, choices, or priorities*

Initial response: "I appreciate that you want to help me optimize this. I'm going to handle it according to my priorities."

If they persist: "I can see you have ideas about better approaches. I'm making this decision based on what matters to me."

If they continue: "I understand you see opportunities for improvement. I'm choosing my path."

Template 10: Expertise assertion *Situation: Your partner emphasizes their superior knowledge or experience*

Initial response: "You definitely know more about this than I do, and I'm choosing to learn through my own experience."

If they persist: "I appreciate your expertise. I want to try my approach and see how it works."

If they continue: "I understand you have more knowledge in this area. I'm comfortable with my current understanding."

Each template follows the same pattern: acknowledge their perspective, maintain your choice, and avoid getting pulled into debates about whose approach is objectively better. Practice these responses until they feel natural, so you can use them automatically during actual conflicts.

Building collaboration without losing autonomy

The goal of these communication strategies isn't to shut down all input from your partner or create rigid separation between your choices. The goal is to create space for genuine collaboration based on mutual respect rather than one person's standards dominating all decisions.

Once you've established that you have autonomy over your own choices, you can begin inviting your partner's expertise in ways that feel supportive rather than controlling.

Structured input requests give you control over when and how you receive suggestions:

- "I'm working on this project and would love your thoughts once I get to the research phase."

- "I'd appreciate your expertise on the technical aspects of this decision after I narrow down my preferences."

- "Could you help me brainstorm alternatives for this situation I'm trying to solve?"

Collaborative planning involves both people contributing to decisions while maintaining individual areas of control:

- "Let's each research different aspects of this trip and then combine our findings."

- "What if you handle the budget analysis and I focus on the lifestyle factors we should consider?"

- "Can we divide this project so you optimize the efficiency elements and I handle the creative aspects?"

Optional consultation makes it clear that input is welcome but not required:

- "I'm making this decision on my own, but if you have quick thoughts, I'm happy to hear them."

- "I don't need help with this, but if you notice anything important I should consider, feel free to mention it."

- "I've got this handled, but you're welcome to share any relevant information you come across."

Appreciation for expertise acknowledges your partner's knowledge while maintaining your decision-making authority:

- "I really value your analytical skills. When I want that kind of input, you're the person I'll ask."

- "You're incredibly good at finding optimal solutions. I appreciate knowing I can tap into that expertise when I need it."

- "I love that you're so thorough in your research. It's really helpful when I'm facing complex decisions."

This balanced approach allows you to benefit from your partner's strengths without feeling overwhelmed by their standards or losing your sense of competence and autonomy.

Creating emotional safety for authentic communication

OCPD relationships often develop patterns where conversations become debates about methods, approaches, and optimal outcomes. This can make it difficult to share feelings, concerns, or preferences that might not align with your partner's analytical framework.

Creating emotional safety requires establishing that feelings and preferences are valid data points even when they don't fit logical optimization models.

Emotional validity statements establish that feelings matter regardless of whether they're logical:

- "I know this feeling might not make logical sense, and it's important to me."

- "I understand you see this differently, and this is how the situation feels to me."

- "I can see why you'd analyze it that way, and my emotional response is still valid information."

Preference protection maintains your right to choices based on personal factors rather than objective criteria:

- "I know there are more efficient options, and I prefer this one for personal reasons."

- "I understand this isn't the optimal choice, and it feels right to me."

- "I can see the logic in your alternative, and I'm drawn to this option for reasons I can't fully explain."

Process requests ask for specific types of communication that support emotional connection:

- "I'd like to share how I'm feeling about this situation. I'm not looking for solutions right now, just understanding."

- "Can we talk about this without focusing on what the best approach would be? I just want you to understand my perspective."

- "I want to tell you about my experience with this. I'm not asking you to agree, just to listen."

Curiosity invitations encourage your partner to be interested in your perspective without immediately jumping to optimization:

- "I'm wondering if you'd like to understand why this approach appeals to me."

- "Would you be interested in hearing about what matters to me in this situation?"

- "I'd love to share what I'm considering as I think through this decision."

These communication approaches help your partner understand that not all conversations are problem-solving sessions. Sometimes the goal is connection, understanding, or simply sharing experiences without needing to optimize outcomes.

Navigating the improvement without invalidation balance

One of the most delicate aspects of OCPD communication is helping your partner understand that you can appreciate their expertise while still choosing different approaches. This balance requires acknowledging their superior knowledge in some areas while maintaining your right to prioritize factors beyond optimization.

Your partner's suggestions often are improvements from a technical standpoint. Their restaurant recommendations usually are better reviewed. Their organizational systems usually are more efficient. Their research usually does reveal superior options.

The issue isn't whether their suggestions have merit—it's about creating space for other priorities and decision-making approaches that don't always prioritize optimal outcomes.

Merit acknowledgment without adoption lets you recognize good advice without feeling obligated to follow it:

- "That's really excellent research, and I'm choosing convenience over value for this purchase."

- "You've identified genuinely better options, and I'm satisfied with my choice."

- "I can see why that approach would produce superior results, and I prefer my method for this situation."

Values clarification helps your partner understand that you're making intentional choices based on different priorities:

- "I know efficiency is really important to you, and spontaneity matters more to me for this decision."

- "I understand you prioritize optimal outcomes, and I'm balancing multiple factors including how much energy I want to spend on this."

- "I can see you value thorough preparation, and I prefer learning as I go for this particular situation."

Expertise appreciation reinforces that you respect their knowledge while maintaining your autonomy:

- "I really appreciate how much you know about this topic. I'm making this choice based on my personal priorities."

- "Your expertise in this area is impressive, and I'm choosing a simpler approach that works for my current needs."

- "I value your analytical skills tremendously, and I want to trust my instincts on this decision."

This communication style helps your partner understand that rejecting their suggestions isn't about rejecting their competence or value. You're simply choosing to prioritize different factors in your decision-making process.

Specific language that reduces defensiveness and promotes cooperation

The communication strategies in this chapter work because they address your partner's core need to have their expertise acknowledged while protecting your need for autonomy and decision-making authority. They reduce defensiveness because they don't attack your partner's competence or suggest their methods are wrong. Instead, they create parallel validity where both approaches can coexist.

These techniques promote cooperation because they transform either/or conflicts into both/and collaborations. Instead of debating whose approach is superior, you acknowledge that multiple approaches can have merit while maintaining your right to choose based on your own priorities and preferences.

The key insight is that OCPD partners don't need you to adopt their methods, but they do need recognition that their methods have value. Once that recognition is provided, many OCPD partners can relax their persuasion efforts and allow you to proceed according to your own preferences.

This doesn't solve every communication challenge in OCPD relationships, but it eliminates many of the recurring conflicts that exhaust both partners and allows more energy to be directed toward connection, appreciation, and genuine collaboration on shared goals.

Chapter 6: Protecting your mental health when nothing is ever good enough

Maria sat in her car after grocery shopping, staring at her carefully organized list with color-coded categories and backup options for each item. She'd followed her husband Roberto's optimization system perfectly—grouping items by store layout, checking for sales, comparing unit prices. The trip had been efficient and cost-effective.

So why did she feel like crying?

The answer hit her as she watched other shoppers casually tossing items into their carts, chatting on their phones, picking up impulse purchases without consulting detailed research. She couldn't recall the last time she'd bought something spontaneously or made a simple decision without anticipating Roberto's analysis of why a different choice would have been better.

She'd become efficient, organized, and thorough. She'd also lost something essential—the ability to trust her own instincts and feel confident in her choices, even simple ones like which brand of pasta to buy.

Maria's grocery store revelation isn't unusual for partners in OCPD relationships. The constant exposure to optimization pressure doesn't just change your behavior—it changes how you think about yourself and your capabilities. You may find yourself second-guessing decisions you used to make confidently, feeling anxious about tasks that used to feel routine, or losing touch with your own preferences in favor of objectively "better" options.

This mental health impact is insidious because it happens gradually. Each individual correction or improvement seems reasonable and helpful. The cumulative effect, however, can be a significant erosion of self-confidence, decision-making ability, and personal autonomy.

Protecting your mental health in an OCPD relationship requires **active, intentional strategies** that preserve your sense of competence and personal authority while navigating your partner's need for control and optimization.

Daily self-care protocols for emotional depletion

Living with someone who has OCPD creates a specific type of emotional drain that requires targeted self-care strategies. Traditional self-care advice often focuses on relaxation and stress reduction, but OCPD relationships require approaches that actively rebuild your confidence, autonomy, and sense of personal competence.

Morning autonomy rituals help you start each day from your own center rather than immediately adapting to your partner's standards:

Personal decision practice: Make at least three small decisions each morning based purely on your preferences—what to wear, what to have for breakfast, which route to take to work. Notice how these choices feel when you're not consulting anyone else or optimizing for anything beyond what you want.

Confidence affirmations: Spend five minutes acknowledging your competence: "I make good decisions based on what I know and what matters to me." "My approach to tasks is valid and effective." "I have good judgment about my own life."

Preference checking: Ask yourself what you actually want or prefer for the day ahead, before considering anyone else's opinions or suggestions. What would make you feel happy, energized, or satisfied?

Midday boundary reinforcement helps you maintain your sense of autonomy throughout the day:

Choice celebration: Notice and appreciate moments when you've made decisions or approached tasks according to your own judgment. Give yourself credit for maintaining your autonomy, even in small ways.

Pressure relief: If you've been feeling overwhelmed by your partner's standards or suggestions, take five minutes to remind yourself: "I can appreciate their expertise while trusting my own judgment." "Different approaches can both be valid." "I don't have to optimize every decision to be a capable person."

Energy assessment: Check in with your emotional state. Are you feeling competent and autonomous, or are you starting to feel overwhelmed by external expectations? Adjust your boundaries accordingly.

Evening restoration practices help you recover from the emotional labor of navigating OCPD dynamics:

Accomplishment recognition: Identify at least three things you handled well during the day, regardless of whether they were done optimally. Focus on your effort, decision-making, and follow-through rather than perfect outcomes.

Preference reclamation: Engage in an activity that reflects your personal taste or style rather than optimized outcomes. Listen to music you enjoy (not necessarily the "best" music), watch shows that entertain you, wear clothes that make you feel good.

Emotional processing: Spend time acknowledging any feelings of frustration, inadequacy, or exhaustion without trying to fix or improve them. Your emotions are valid responses to challenging relationship dynamics.

Research shows that partners of individuals with personality disorders benefit significantly from structured self-care practices that specifically address the unique stressors of these relationships (Lavner et al., 2018). The key is consistency rather than intensity—

small daily practices that preserve your sense of self are more effective than occasional large self-care efforts.

Cognitive strategies to counter internalized criticism

One of the most damaging aspects of OCPD relationships is the gradual internalization of your partner's critical voice. Over time, you may find yourself automatically evaluating your choices through their lens, anticipating their improvements, or feeling inadequate when you don't meet their standards.

Cognitive strategies help you recognize when this internal criticism is happening and replace it with more balanced, self-supportive thinking.

Critical voice recognition helps you identify when your partner's standards have become your internal dialogue:

Watch for thoughts like:

- "I should have researched this more thoroughly"
- "There's probably a better way to do this"
- "I'm being lazy/careless/inefficient"
- "I should know how to do this correctly"
- "This isn't good enough"

These thoughts often reflect your partner's values and standards rather than your own authentic assessment of the situation.

Voice separation techniques help you distinguish between your authentic self-assessment and internalized OCPD criticism:

Whose standards are these? When you notice self-critical thoughts, ask: "Am I evaluating this based on my own priorities, or am I using my partner's criteria for what's acceptable?"

What would I tell a friend? If a friend approached a similar situation the way you did, what would you say to them? This often reveals more compassionate and realistic assessment than the critical voice provides.

Historical perspective: How did you evaluate similar situations before your relationship? What standards felt reasonable and motivating to you before being exposed to OCPD optimization pressure?

Cognitive reframing replaces harsh internal criticism with balanced, supportive self-talk:

Instead of: "I should have done this better." **Try:** "I handled this appropriately given my priorities and available energy."

Instead of: "I'm being careless/lazy." **Try:** "I'm choosing efficiency over perfection, and that's a valid choice."

Instead of: "This isn't good enough." **Try:** "This meets my needs and standards, even if it's not optimal."

Instead of: "I should have researched this more." **Try:** "I made this decision with reasonable information and good judgment."

Instead of: "I'm doing this wrong." **Try:** "I'm doing this my way, which is different from but not inferior to other approaches."

Competence reinforcement actively builds evidence for your capability and good judgment:

Daily competence journaling: Write down three decisions you made or tasks you completed successfully each day, focusing on your problem-solving, judgment, and follow-through rather than perfect outcomes.

Historical success review: Regularly remind yourself of past situations where your approach worked well, decisions that turned out positively, and problems you solved effectively.

Strength identification: Make a list of your natural abilities, preferred approaches, and areas of competence. Refer to this list when you're feeling inadequate or incompetent.

Feedback balance: Actively seek input from people other than your partner about your capabilities, judgment, and approaches. This provides perspective on your competence that isn't filtered through OCPD standards.

Building your support network despite their disapproval

OCPD partners often have strong opinions about social activities, friend choices, and time management that can gradually isolate you from your support network. They may not forbid social connections, but their concerns about efficiency, optimal time use, or the wisdom of your social choices can create subtle pressure to reduce outside relationships.

Building and maintaining supportive connections despite this pressure is crucial for your mental health and perspective.

Friendship maintenance strategies help you preserve relationships that provide emotional support and reality-checking:

Direct communication: Let close friends know that you may need extra patience or flexibility as you navigate some relationship challenges. You don't need to share details, but acknowledging that you're dealing with some stress can help friends understand if you're less available or seem different.

Individual activities: Maintain friendships through activities that don't require your partner's participation or approval. Coffee dates, phone calls, individual hobbies, or one-on-one activities are less likely to trigger your partner's social optimization concerns.

Boundary language with partner: When your partner expresses concerns about your social choices, use the communication techniques from the previous chapter: "I can see you think there might be more productive uses of my time, and maintaining friendships is important to my well-being."

Energy management: Accept that social activities might require more emotional energy than they used to, since you may need to manage your partner's concerns or opinions about your choices. Plan accordingly and don't overcommit.

Professional support development provides objective perspective on your relationship dynamics:

Individual therapy: Working with a therapist who understands personality disorders can provide invaluable support for maintaining your mental health and developing effective strategies. Look for therapists experienced with OCPD relationships.

Support groups: Online or in-person groups for partners of people with personality disorders can provide validation, practical strategies, and connection with others who understand your experience.

Medical support: If you're experiencing depression, anxiety, or other mental health symptoms, professional treatment can help you maintain emotional stability while working on relationship dynamics.

Spiritual or philosophical support: Whether through religious communities, meditation groups, or philosophical exploration, having perspectives that help you maintain your sense of self and values can be crucial.

Family relationship navigation requires special attention when your partner has strong opinions about family interactions:

Separate visits: Maintain individual relationships with family members through calls, visits, or activities that don't require your partner's participation.

Information boundaries: You don't need to share your partner's critiques or suggestions about family members, and you don't need to defend your family's approaches to your partner.

Holiday negotiations: Develop strategies for managing family gatherings and holidays that honor both your need for family connection and your partner's need for structure and planning.

Conflict prevention: Avoid situations where your family members and partner are likely to clash over different approaches to tasks, decisions, or standards.

Emergency self-care plan for crisis moments

OCPD relationships can create intense moments of feeling overwhelmed, inadequate, or trapped by impossible standards. Having a prepared emergency self-care plan helps you manage these crisis moments without making impulsive decisions that could damage your relationship or your well-being.

Crisis recognition signs help you identify when you need immediate self-care intervention:

Emotional indicators:

- Feeling like you can't do anything right
- Overwhelming urge to escape or run away
- Intense anger or resentment toward your partner
- Complete loss of confidence in your judgment
- Feeling like you're disappearing or losing yourself

Physical indicators:

- Panic symptoms (racing heart, difficulty breathing, sweating)
- Exhaustion that sleep doesn't relieve
- Tension headaches or muscle pain
- Changes in appetite or sleep patterns
- Feeling physically sick when anticipating interactions with your partner

Behavioral indicators:

- Avoiding tasks because you fear criticism
- Asking for permission for decisions you used to make independently
- Constantly second-guessing your choices
- Isolating from friends and activities you used to enjoy
- Finding yourself adopting your partner's critical voice toward others

Immediate crisis interventions provide quick relief when you're feeling overwhelmed:

Physical grounding:

- Step outside for fresh air and change of environment
- Take five deep breaths focusing only on the sensation of breathing
- Do brief physical exercise to release tension and anxiety
- Take a hot shower or bath to reset your nervous system

Mental reset:

- Remind yourself: "My partner's standards are not the only valid standards"
- Say aloud: "I am a competent person who makes reasonable decisions"
- List three things you've handled well recently, regardless of whether they were optimal
- Call or text someone who appreciates you for who you are

Emotional regulation:

- Allow yourself to feel frustrated, angry, or sad without trying to fix these emotions
- Write down your feelings without censoring or analyzing them
- Give yourself permission to temporarily avoid your partner while you regain equilibrium
- Remind yourself that your emotional reactions are valid responses to difficult circumstances

Short-term protection strategies help you create space while you recover from crisis moments:

Temporary boundaries:

- "I need some time to myself right now"
- "I'm going to handle this without input for now"
- "I need a break from discussing methods and approaches"
- "I'm not available for suggestions about this topic today"

Environmental changes:

- Spend time in spaces your partner doesn't control or optimize
- Engage in activities that reflect your taste and preferences
- Listen to music, watch shows, or read books your partner wouldn't choose
- Visit places that make you feel relaxed and confident

Support activation:

- Reach out to friends or family members who remind you of your competence
- Contact your therapist if you have one, or consider finding professional support

- Connect with online communities for partners of people with personality disorders
- Schedule time with people who appreciate your natural approach to life

Self-Care Assessment and Planning Worksheet

Regular assessment of your mental health and self-care needs helps you maintain perspective and identify areas that need attention before they become crisis situations.

Current Mental Health Assessment

Rate each area from 1 (very poor) to 10 (excellent):

Confidence in your own judgment: ___ What specific situations make you doubt yourself most?

Energy levels throughout the day: ___ When do you feel most drained, and what seems to trigger that drain?

Ability to maintain your own preferences: ___ In what areas do you find yourself automatically adopting your partner's standards?

Connection to supportive relationships: ___ How often do you have meaningful interactions with people other than your partner?

Sense of personal autonomy: ___ What decisions do you make independently vs. what requires input or approval?

Emotional stability and resilience: ___ How well are you managing stress, frustration, and challenging emotions?

Physical health and energy: ___ Are you experiencing physical symptoms of stress or emotional strain?

Overall life satisfaction: ___ How satisfied are you with your life outside of relationship challenges?

Priority Self-Care Areas

Based on your assessment, identify the three areas that need most attention:

Priority 1: ___ **Current challenge:** ___ **Specific self-care goals:** ___ **Daily practices that could help:** ___ **Weekly practices that could help:** ___ **Monthly practices that could help:** ___

Priority 2: ___ **Current challenge:** ___ **Specific self-care goals:** ___ **Daily practices that could help:** ___ **Weekly practices that could help:** ___ **Monthly practices that could help:** ___

Priority 3: ___ **Current challenge:** ___ **Specific self-care goals:** ___ **Daily practices that could help:** ___ **Weekly practices that could help:** ___ **Monthly practices that could help:** ___

Support System Mapping

People who provide emotional support: ___ **People who remind you of your competence:** ___ **People who share your values and approaches:** ___ **Professional support you currently have:** ___ **Professional support you might benefit from:** ___

Emergency Support Plan

Crisis warning signs specific to you: ___

People to contact during crisis moments: ___

Activities that help you regain perspective: ___

Places you can go for emotional reset: ___

Phrases or reminders that help during difficult moments: ___

Self-Care Commitment

Daily practices you commit to maintaining: ___

Weekly practices you commit to implementing: ___

Monthly assessment and adjustment schedule: ___

Boundaries you need to maintain for your mental health: ___

Signs that indicate you need professional support: ___

This assessment should be repeated every three months or whenever you notice significant changes in your mental health or relationship dynamics.

Rebuilding confidence in your own judgment

One of the most important aspects of mental health protection in OCPD relationships is actively rebuilding and maintaining confidence in your own decision-making abilities. Constant exposure to optimization pressure can erode your trust in your own judgment, even in areas where you have expertise and good instincts.

Decision-making practice helps you rebuild confidence through intentional choices:

Start small: Make several low-stakes decisions each day based purely on your preferences without seeking input or validation. Choose your lunch, your route to work, your weekend activities based on what you want rather than what's optimal.

Document successes: Keep track of decisions that work out well, problems you solve effectively, and situations you handle competently. This creates evidence that counters the narrative that your judgment is inadequate.

Accept imperfection: Practice making decisions that are "good enough" rather than optimal, and notice that most suboptimal choices don't create significant problems or consequences.

Trust your expertise: In areas where you have knowledge, experience, or natural ability, practice making decisions without extensive research or outside input. Notice how your competence feels when it's not being filtered through someone else's standards.

Intuition development helps you reconnect with your natural decision-making process:

Body awareness: Pay attention to how different choices feel physically. Your body often provides good information about what works for you, separate from analytical optimization.

Initial instincts: Notice your first response to decisions before you start analyzing all the alternatives. This initial instinct often reflects your authentic preferences and values.

Energy monitoring: Choose options that feel energizing rather than depleting, even when the energizing choice isn't the most efficient or optimal.

Value alignment: Make decisions based on what matters to you personally rather than what produces the best objective outcomes. Your values are valid criteria for decision-making.

Creating sustainable mental health practices

Protecting your mental health in an OCPD relationship isn't a temporary project—it's an ongoing practice that needs to be sustainable over the long term. This means developing approaches that don't require enormous amounts of time or energy but still provide consistent support for your well-being.

Integrated self-care builds mental health protection into your daily routine rather than adding it as extra tasks:

Mindful moments: Use routine activities (brushing teeth, drinking coffee, commuting) as opportunities to check in with yourself and appreciate your autonomy.

Preference honoring: Look for small ways throughout each day to honor your preferences and tastes rather than always optimizing for efficiency or quality.

Competence acknowledgment: Get in the habit of noticing when you handle situations well, make good decisions, or solve problems effectively, regardless of whether the outcome was optimal.

Boundary maintenance: Incorporate boundary-setting language into your regular communication so it becomes natural rather than a special effort.

Long-term resilience building develops your capacity to maintain mental health despite ongoing relationship challenges:

Identity preservation: Maintain interests, activities, and relationships that reflect who you are separate from your partner's influence or optimization.

Personal growth: Pursue learning, development, and new experiences that build confidence and expand your sense of competence.

Future planning: Maintain goals and plans that are yours alone, whether or not your partner shares or optimizes them.

Professional development: Build skills, expertise, and accomplishments that give you confidence in your abilities outside your relationship.

Support system investment: Continue building relationships that provide perspective, appreciation, and reality-checking about your capabilities and worth.

Recognizing when professional help is needed

While self-care strategies are essential, there are times when professional support becomes necessary for managing the mental health impacts of OCPD relationships. Recognizing these signs early can prevent more serious mental health deterioration.

Signs that indicate need for professional support:

Depression indicators:

- Persistent feelings of hopelessness or worthlessness
- Loss of interest in activities you previously enjoyed

- Significant changes in sleep or appetite patterns
- Difficulty concentrating on work or daily tasks
- Thoughts of self-harm or that life isn't worth living

Anxiety symptoms:

- Panic attacks or overwhelming fear about daily decisions
- Constant worry about doing things "wrong" or disappointing your partner
- Physical symptoms like rapid heartbeat, sweating, or difficulty breathing
- Avoidance of tasks or situations due to fear of criticism
- Hypervigilance about your partner's reactions or moods

Identity confusion:

- Inability to remember what you used to enjoy or prefer
- Feeling like you don't know who you are outside your partner's expectations
- Complete loss of confidence in your own judgment
- Feeling like you're becoming someone you don't recognize
- Inability to make decisions without extensive anxiety

Relationship deterioration:

- Increasing resentment toward your partner despite their good intentions
- Fantasy about escape or ending the relationship as the only solution
- Complete shutdown of communication to avoid conflict
- Loss of all emotional and physical intimacy

- Feeling trapped with no viable options for improvement

Professional support options provide different types of assistance depending on your specific needs:

Individual therapy helps you process your experiences, develop coping strategies, and maintain your sense of self. Look for therapists with experience in personality disorders, codependency, or relationship trauma.

Couples therapy can be beneficial if your partner is willing to participate and the therapist understands OCPD dynamics. However, individual therapy is often recommended first to help you establish boundaries and clarity.

Psychiatric evaluation may be helpful if you're experiencing depression, anxiety, or other mental health symptoms that could benefit from medication support.

Support groups (in-person or online) connect you with others facing similar challenges and provide validation that your experiences are real and understandable.

The decision to seek professional help doesn't mean you've failed or that your relationship is hopeless. It means you're taking responsibility for your mental health and getting the support you need to navigate a challenging situation effectively.

Building hope without minimizing reality

Protecting your mental health in an OCPD relationship requires balancing realistic acknowledgment of the challenges with hope for improvement and growth. This isn't about toxic positivity or pretending everything is fine—it's about maintaining perspective on what's possible while taking care of yourself.

Realistic hope focuses on what can actually change:

Your responses to your partner's behavior can become more effective and less emotionally draining as you develop better strategies and boundaries.

Your confidence in your own judgment and capabilities can be rebuilt and maintained despite ongoing exposure to optimization pressure.

Your support systems can be strengthened to provide perspective and validation outside your relationship.

Your self-care practices can become more effective at protecting your mental health and maintaining your sense of self.

Your partner's awareness of how their behavior affects you can sometimes improve, especially with professional support.

Your relationship dynamics can shift toward more balance and mutual respect, even if your partner's basic OCPD traits don't change.

Unrealistic hope that can lead to disappointment and further mental health challenges:

Expecting your partner to suddenly become flexible, spontaneous, or comfortable with suboptimal outcomes. Their brain is wired differently, and these changes don't happen quickly or easily.

Believing that if you just explain your feelings clearly enough, your partner will understand and change their behavior. OCPD affects how they process information about efficiency and optimization.

Thinking that your partner's behavior will improve without active effort and often professional support from both of you.

Assuming that love and good intentions are enough to overcome the challenges that OCPD creates in relationships.

Sustainable hope is based on gradual progress, increased understanding, and improved coping strategies rather than dramatic transformation. Many couples do find ways to create more balanced, satisfying relationships while managing OCPD challenges, but this happens through consistent effort over time rather than sudden breakthroughs.

Your mental health matters regardless of whether your relationship improves. Taking care of yourself isn't selfish—it's necessary for your well-being and for your ability to participate in any relationship in a healthy way.

The goal isn't to eliminate all stress or challenge from your relationship. The goal is to maintain your sense of self, your confidence in your own judgment, and your overall mental health while navigating the unique challenges that OCPD relationships create.

You deserve to feel competent, valued, and emotionally stable in your relationship. If your current situation doesn't support these basic needs, seeking help and making changes isn't giving up on your relationship—it's taking responsibility for your own well-being and creating the conditions where a healthier relationship might become possible.

Comprehensive mental health protection strategies

The strategies in this chapter work together to create a comprehensive approach to protecting your mental health while living with someone whose brain is wired for constant optimization and control. They acknowledge that OCPD creates unique stresses that require specific responses rather than generic self-care advice.

The daily practices help you maintain your sense of autonomy and competence on an ongoing basis. The cognitive strategies protect you from internalizing your partner's critical voice. The support system development ensures you have perspective and validation outside your relationship. The emergency protocols help you manage crisis moments without making impulsive decisions.

Most importantly, these strategies recognize that your mental health is your responsibility and your priority. You can't control your partner's OCPD symptoms, but you can control how you respond to them and how well you take care of yourself in the process.

This isn't about becoming selfish or uncaring toward your partner. It's about maintaining enough emotional and mental stability to participate in your relationship from a position of strength rather than depletion. When you take care of your own mental health, you're better able to respond to your partner's challenges with compassion rather than resentment, and you're more likely to make thoughtful decisions about your relationship based on clear thinking rather than emotional overwhelm.

Your mental health matters. Your needs are legitimate. Your well-being deserves protection and priority, regardless of how well-intentioned your partner's behavior might be.

Chapter 7: When children are involved

breaking the perfectionist cycle

Eight-year-old Emma sat at the kitchen table, tears streaming down her face as she erased her math homework for the fourth time. The numbers were neat enough. Her work was correct. But somehow, it still wasn't meeting her father's standards for proper presentation.

"See how the 7 looks different from the other 7s?" David pointed to her paper. "If you keep them all the same size and angle, your teacher will be able to see how careful you are with your work."

Emma's mother, Sarah, watched from the doorway feeling helpless and increasingly angry. This homework session had already lasted two hours. Emma had solved every problem correctly on the first try, but the rewriting for "neatness improvement" had turned routine homework into an exhausting perfectionist marathon.

"David," Sarah said quietly, "she's eight years old. The homework is finished and correct."

"I just want her to develop good habits," David replied, genuinely confused by Sarah's concern. "Attention to detail will serve her well throughout her life."

But Emma wasn't learning attention to detail. She was learning that her best effort wasn't good enough, that completing tasks correctly wasn't sufficient, and that adult approval required meeting impossibly high standards. Most concerning of all, she was beginning to show signs of anxiety about starting her homework, knowing it would never be finished quickly or easily.

This scene plays out in thousands of households where one parent has OCPD. The parent genuinely wants to help their child succeed and develop good habits. But their disorder creates standards and expectations that are developmentally inappropriate and emotionally harmful for children.

Protecting children from the negative impacts of OCPD while preserving family stability and the positive aspects of the OCPD parent's contribution requires careful navigation, clear boundaries, and age-appropriate strategies that shield kids from impossible standards.

Understanding how OCPD affects children differently at various stages

OCPD impacts children differently depending on their developmental stage, temperament, and the specific ways the condition manifests in their parent. Understanding these variations helps you provide appropriate protection and support.

Early childhood (ages 2-6) impacts:

Young children are naturally messy, impulsive, and learning basic skills through trial and error. OCPD parents may struggle with the chaos and inefficiency that's normal and necessary for healthy child development.

Common OCPD parent responses:

- Cleaning up children's play areas while they're still playing
- Correcting how children hold crayons, use scissors, or complete simple tasks
- Becoming anxious when children make normal messes during learning
- Insisting on specific routines and methods for basic self-care tasks

- Having difficulty with the unpredictability of young children's needs and schedules

Potential impacts on children:

- Reduced willingness to explore and experiment if messes create parental anxiety

- Premature pressure to master skills before they're developmentally ready

- Anxiety about making mistakes or getting things "wrong"

- Difficulty developing independence if parents take over tasks frequently

- Reduced spontaneity and natural playfulness

School age (ages 6-12) impacts:

School-age children are developing academic skills, social relationships, and personal interests. OCPD parents may focus intensely on academic performance and organization while struggling with children's need for social play and creative exploration.

Common OCPD parent responses:

- Excessive involvement in homework completion and presentation

- Criticism of teachers' standards as too low or inconsistent

- Difficulty with children's interest in activities that seem "wasteful" or inefficient

- Pressure to excel in all academic areas rather than developing natural strengths

- Anxiety about children's social choices and time management

Potential impacts on children:

- Homework anxiety and procrastination due to perfectionist pressure

- Reduced confidence in their own academic abilities

- Social difficulties if parental standards conflict with peer norms

- Loss of interest in creative activities that don't have clear "right" answers

- Premature focus on achievement rather than learning and exploration

Adolescence (ages 13-18) impacts:

Teenagers naturally push boundaries, make mistakes, and develop independence. OCPD parents may struggle intensely with their adolescent's need to make decisions without extensive research and optimization.

Common OCPD parent responses:

- Detailed analysis of teenagers' social choices and friend selections

- Difficulty accepting normal teenage mistakes as learning experiences

- Pressure to optimize college preparation and extracurricular activities

- Conflict over teenagers' different values and priorities

- Anxiety about teenagers' increasing independence and decision-making

Potential impacts on teenagers:

- Rebellion against all standards rather than developing healthy personal standards

- Difficulty making decisions independently due to over-involvement from parent

- Resentment toward parental criticism and optimization attempts

- Anxiety about disappointing parents with normal teenage choices

- Identity confusion about personal values versus parental expectations

Individual temperament differences also affect how children respond to OCPD parenting:

Naturally organized children may initially thrive under OCPD parenting but later struggle with anxiety and rigid thinking patterns that limit their flexibility and creativity.

Creative, spontaneous children often feel more immediate stress from OCPD standards but may also develop better boundaries and self-advocacy skills in response.

Sensitive children may internalize OCPD criticism deeply and develop anxiety, perfectionism, or depression at higher rates.

Strong-willed children may engage in more direct conflict with OCPD parents but also maintain better sense of personal autonomy.

Understanding your specific child's temperament and developmental stage helps you provide appropriate support and protection while working with their natural personality rather than against it.

Protecting children from impossible standards

The most crucial aspect of co-parenting with an OCPD partner is protecting children from developmentally inappropriate expectations while maintaining family harmony and respect for both parents.

Age-appropriate expectation advocacy involves helping your OCPD partner understand what's realistic for children at different developmental stages:

For young children: "At age four, she's still learning how to hold scissors correctly. Expecting perfect cutting technique creates frustration rather than skill development."

For school-age children: "Third-graders typically need 20-30 minutes for homework like this. Spending two hours on presentation details takes away from family time and creates negative associations with learning."

For teenagers: "Making some poor decisions is how teenagers learn judgment. Our job is to keep them safe and provide guidance, not prevent all mistakes."

Intervention strategies help you step in when OCPD standards become harmful without undermining your partner's parental authority:

Time limits: "Let's set a 30-minute limit for homework help. If it's not finished by then, we'll send a note to the teacher about the difficulty level."

Good enough standards: "This meets the assignment requirements. Extra improvements are optional, not necessary."

Developmental reminders: "She's learning this skill for the first time. Mistakes and imperfection are part of the process."

Break provision: "I can see you're both getting frustrated. Let's take a break and come back to this in 15 minutes."

Alternative approaches: "What if we try a different method that might work better for how her brain learns?"

Child advocacy phrases help you support your child's needs without directly criticizing your partner:

- "I think she's done enough work on this for tonight"

- "Let's celebrate that he completed the assignment correctly"

- "She seems to be getting overwhelmed by all the corrections"

- "What if we focus on one improvement area instead of several?"

- "I want to make sure this stays fun and positive for her"

The key is positioning yourself as an advocate for your child's developmental needs rather than an opponent of your partner's standards.

Age-appropriate explanations of parent's behavior

Children need help understanding why one parent has very high standards and specific ways of doing things. Age-appropriate explanations can reduce children's confusion and self-blame while helping them develop healthy responses to perfectionist pressure.

For young children (ages 4-7):

"Daddy's brain likes things to be very neat and organized. That's just how he thinks, and it doesn't mean you're doing anything wrong when things get messy. Some people like things very tidy, and some people are okay with more mess. Both ways are fine."

"Mommy wants to help you do your best work, and sometimes she gives so many suggestions that it feels overwhelming. You can tell me if you're feeling frustrated, and we can take breaks when you need them."

"Some parents worry more about mistakes than others. When Papa seems upset about small things, it's because he cares about helping you learn, not because you did something bad."

For school-age children (ages 8-12):

"Dad has something called perfectionism, which means his brain notices when things could be done better or more carefully. This can be helpful sometimes, but it can also make regular activities feel stressful. His perfectionism is about how his brain works, not about whether you're doing good work."

"Mom has very high standards because she wants good outcomes for our family. Sometimes her standards are higher than what's really necessary, and that's not your fault. You're learning, and learning involves making mistakes and doing things imperfectly while you practice."

"When a parent focuses a lot on how things are done instead of celebrating that they got done, it can make you feel like nothing you do is good enough. That feeling comes from their perfectionism, not from any problems with your work or effort."

For teenagers (ages 13-18):

"Your mom has OCPD, which affects how she thinks about efficiency, standards, and the 'right' way to do things. She genuinely believes her approaches are better, and she offers suggestions because she wants good outcomes for you. You can appreciate her expertise while also developing your own judgment about what matters to you."

"Dad's brain is wired to see opportunities for improvement everywhere. This makes him excellent at problem-solving and achieving high-quality results, but it can also make him critical of approaches that work fine but aren't optimal. His criticism usually isn't about you personally—it's about his discomfort with inefficiency."

"Living with a perfectionist parent can make you feel like you're constantly being evaluated. That's a real challenge, and it's not something you caused or can fix by being more perfect. Your job is to develop your own sense of what's good enough while respecting your parent's different standards."

Teaching children response strategies helps them maintain their self-esteem while navigating perfectionist pressure:

For all ages:

- "You can say 'I'm proud of my work' when someone suggests improvements you don't want to make"
- "It's okay to take breaks when perfectionist pressure feels overwhelming"
- "You can ask for help if suggestions are making you feel bad about your work"

For older children:

- "You can appreciate someone's expertise without adopting all their standards"
- "Different people have different ideas about what's good enough, and both can be right"
- "You can thank someone for suggestions and still choose your own approach"

The goal is helping children understand that perfectionist behavior is about the parent's condition, not about the child's inadequacy or failure to meet reasonable standards.

Building children's resilience and self-esteem

Children living with perfectionist parents need extra support developing confidence in their own judgment, tolerance for imperfection, and resilience when facing criticism or impossible standards.

Confidence building activities help children maintain self-esteem despite exposure to constant optimization pressure:

Effort celebration: Focus praise on children's effort, persistence, and improvement rather than perfect outcomes. "I'm proud of how hard you worked on this" carries more weight than "This is perfect."

Process appreciation: Notice and comment on children's problem-solving approaches, creativity, and independent thinking. "I like how you figured out a different way to solve that problem."

Mistake normalization: Share stories about your own mistakes and learning experiences. Help children understand that errors are information rather than failures.

Personal strength recognition: Help children identify their natural talents, preferred learning styles, and unique approaches to tasks and challenges.

Choice validation: Support children's preferences and decisions in age-appropriate areas, even when they differ from what adults might choose.

Resilience development teaches children how to bounce back from criticism and maintain perspective on perfectionist pressure:

Emotional vocabulary: Help children identify and name their feelings when facing perfectionist pressure. "It sounds like you're feeling frustrated that nothing seems good enough."

Coping strategies: Teach specific techniques for managing overwhelm, such as deep breathing, taking breaks, or asking for support.

Perspective skills: Help children distinguish between constructive feedback and perfectionist criticism. "Suggestions that help you learn are different from suggestions that just make things more complicated."

Boundary language: Teach age-appropriate ways to advocate for themselves. "I need a break from suggestions right now" or "I'm satisfied with this work."

Reality checking: Help children understand what's normal for their age group and developmental stage. Connect them with other families where they can see different approaches to standards and expectations.

Self-compassion development helps children maintain kindness toward themselves when facing impossible standards:

Internal dialogue awareness: Help children notice when they're being self-critical and develop kinder ways to talk to themselves about mistakes and imperfection.

Perfectionism recognition: Teach children to recognize when they're adopting impossible standards and help them adjust expectations to more reasonable levels.

Comparison reduction: Help children focus on their own growth and progress rather than comparing themselves to parental standards or other children's achievements.

Enjoyment prioritization: Encourage activities that children find fun and satisfying regardless of whether they produce optimal outcomes.

Identity beyond achievement: Help children develop sense of worth based on who they are rather than what they accomplish or how perfectly they perform.

Co-parenting strategies with an OCPD partner

Successfully co-parenting with an OCPD partner requires strategies that honor their positive contributions while protecting children from harmful aspects of perfectionist parenting.

Division of parental responsibilities can minimize conflicts while maximizing each parent's strengths:

OCPD parent strengths:

- Academic support and homework structure

- Organization systems and planning

- Research for important decisions (schools, activities, medical care)

- Teaching life skills that require precision and attention to detail

- Long-term goal planning and preparation

Non-OCPD parent strengths:

- Emotional support and comfort during struggles

- Creative activities and unstructured play

- Flexibility during changes and unexpected situations

- Social guidance and relationship support

- Stress relief and fun activities

Collaborative areas where both parents contribute:

Major decisions: Both parents provide input, with the OCPD parent handling research and the non-OCPD parent considering emotional and social factors.

Discipline: Develop agreed-upon consequences and approaches that both parents can implement consistently.

School communication: Divide responsibilities so the OCPD parent handles academic concerns while the non-OCPD parent manages social and emotional school issues.

Activity selection: Children participate in activities that reflect both parents' values—some optimized for skill development, others chosen for enjoyment and exploration.

Communication strategies help both parents work together effectively:

Private discussions: Address disagreements about parenting approaches privately rather than in front of children. Present united fronts even when you don't fully agree.

Standards negotiation: "I can see why you want her handwriting to be neater, and I think this level is appropriate for her age. What if we focus on one specific improvement rather than several?"

Time management: "Let's set limits on how long homework help sessions last so they don't take over our entire evening."

Child advocacy: "I'm noticing he's getting frustrated with all the corrections. Can we take a break and celebrate what he's accomplished so far?"

Strength recognition: "You're really good at helping her develop organizational systems. I appreciate how much thought you put into setting her up for success."

Intervention protocols help you step in when perfectionist standards become harmful:

Overwhelm signals: Watch for signs that children are becoming anxious, frustrated, or shutting down due to perfectionist pressure.

Time limits: Establish maximum amounts of time for homework help, chore completion, or other activities that can become perfectionist marathons.

Good enough standards: "This meets the requirements for the assignment. Additional improvements are optional enrichment, not necessary corrections."

Break enforcement: "I can see you're both getting frustrated. Let's pause this activity and return to it later with fresh energy."

Alternative suggestions: "What if we try a different approach that might work better for her learning style?"

Family meeting templates and conversation guides

Regular family meetings can help address perfectionist pressures while maintaining family cohesion and mutual respect. These meetings work best when they follow structured formats that prevent them from becoming criticism or optimization sessions.

Weekly family meeting structure:

Check-in round (10 minutes): Each family member shares one highlight and one challenge from their week without advice or suggestions from others.

Appreciation round (10 minutes): Each person shares something they appreciated about each other family member during the week.

Problem-solving time (15 minutes): Address one specific family issue using structured discussion rather than debate about optimal solutions.

Planning time (10 minutes): Discuss upcoming week's activities, schedules, and any special events or changes.

Fun planning (5 minutes): Plan one enjoyable family activity for the upcoming week that doesn't require optimization or extensive preparation.

Problem-solving conversation guide:

Step 1: Problem identification "The issue we need to address is: _____" "This affects our family because: _____"

Step 2: Multiple perspective sharing Each family member shares their view of the problem without others arguing or correcting their perspective.

Step 3: Solution brainstorming Generate multiple possible solutions without evaluating them initially.

Step 4: Solution evaluation Discuss pros and cons of different approaches, with focus on what works for the whole family rather than what's optimal.

Step 5: Agreement and trial period Choose one approach to try for a specific time period, with plans to reassess and adjust as needed.

Addressing perfectionist pressure in family meetings:

When OCPD parent dominates discussion: "Let's make sure everyone gets equal time to share their thoughts before we start solving the problem."

When suggestions become overwhelming: "We have lots of good ideas. Let's focus on which approach feels workable for everyone."

When children shut down: "I notice some people have gotten quiet. Let's take a break and make sure everyone feels heard."

When standards become the focus: "Our goal is finding something that works for our family, not necessarily finding the perfect solution."

Sample conversation starters for common issues:

Homework stress: "We want to support school success while keeping homework time positive. How can we balance learning with family peace?"

Chore expectations: "Everyone contributes to household tasks, and people have different ways of doing things well. How can we appreciate different approaches?"

Activity planning: "We want family activities that everyone enjoys. How can we balance planning with spontaneity?"

Social situations: "Different families have different styles for social events. How can we respect each other's comfort levels?"

The key is keeping family meetings focused on collaboration and mutual respect rather than allowing them to become forums for perfectionist analysis of family functioning.

Creating buffers between OCPD parent and children

Sometimes the most important parenting strategy is creating space between the OCPD parent and children when perfectionist pressure becomes overwhelming or harmful.

Natural buffer strategies:

Activity division: The non-OCPD parent handles activities that tend to trigger perfectionist responses—creative projects, unstructured play, social situations that require flexibility.

Homework supervision rotation: Alternate who helps with homework, with the OCPD parent focusing on subjects where their expertise is most helpful and the non-OCPD parent handling assignments that need creativity or flexibility.

Bedtime routines: The non-OCPD parent handles bedtime when children need comfort and relaxation rather than optimization of sleep preparation routines.

Morning routines: Divide morning responsibilities so children aren't facing perfectionist pressure when they're tired and need to get ready quickly.

Social events: The non-OCPD parent takes primary responsibility for social interactions that require flexibility and spontaneity.

Crisis intervention strategies:

Emotional overwhelm: "I can see everyone's getting frustrated. Let me take over this activity while Dad takes a break."

Perfectionist escalation: "This seems to be getting stressful for everyone. Let's pause and approach this differently."

Child shutdown: "I think she needs some downtime. Why don't you two spend some time together while I handle this with her?"

Standards conflict: "I know you both want this to be done well. Let's figure out a way that works for everyone."

Time pressure: "We're running out of time for this to stay positive. Let's finish this up and call it good enough for tonight."

Communication with OCPD partner about buffering:

Frame buffering as family optimization rather than criticism of their parenting:

"I notice homework goes more smoothly when we divide it up by subject. You're really good at helping with math, and I seem to work well with her on creative writing."

"The kids seem to respond well when we each handle the activities that match our strengths. You're excellent at skill-building, and I'm good at the emotional support stuff."

"I think we're more effective as a parenting team when we play to our individual strengths rather than both trying to handle everything the same way."

The goal is positioning buffering as strategic family management rather than protection from the OCPD parent.

Teaching children to thrive despite perfectionist pressure

The most important gift you can give children living with an OCPD parent is the ability to maintain their self-esteem, creativity, and confidence despite exposure to impossible standards.

Resilience skills for different ages:

Young children:

- "Your work is good enough when you've tried your best"

- "Mistakes help us learn new things"

- "Different people like things done different ways, and that's okay"

- "You can ask for help if someone's suggestions make you feel bad"

School-age children:

- "Good enough is actually good enough for most things in life"
- "You can appreciate someone's expertise without adopting all their standards"
- "Your effort and learning matter more than perfect results"
- "You have the right to feel proud of your work even if someone sees ways to improve it"

Teenagers:

- "You can develop your own standards based on your values and priorities"
- "Perfectionist pressure often comes from anxiety rather than actual necessity"
- "You can choose when to aim for excellence and when to accept good enough"
- "Your worth isn't determined by how well you meet someone else's standards"

Identity development support:

Personal interest cultivation: Encourage children to pursue activities they enjoy regardless of whether they demonstrate talent or achieve optimal outcomes.

Value clarification: Help children identify what matters to them personally rather than automatically adopting parental priorities.

Decision-making practice: Provide age-appropriate opportunities for children to make choices and experience natural consequences without perfectionist analysis.

Peer connection: Ensure children have opportunities to see how other families approach standards, expectations, and achievement.

Emotional expression: Create safe spaces for children to express frustration, sadness, or anger about perfectionist pressure without having to protect the OCPD parent's feelings.

Future relationship preparation:

Children who grow up with perfectionist parents need specific preparation for healthy adult relationships:

Boundary skills: Teaching children how to maintain their autonomy while respecting others' different approaches.

Perfectionism recognition: Helping children identify when they or others are applying impossible standards to relationships or achievements.

Conflict navigation: Teaching skills for addressing disagreements without trying to prove whose approach is objectively superior.

Self-advocacy: Building confidence in children's ability to express their needs and preferences even when they differ from others' expectations.

Relationship balance: Helping children understand that healthy relationships involve mutual respect rather than one person's standards dominating all decisions.

Breaking generational patterns

One of the most important reasons to address perfectionist pressure in families is preventing these patterns from continuing into the next generation. Children who grow up with impossible standards often develop their own perfectionist tendencies or swing to the opposite extreme of having no standards at all.

Healthy standard development:

Effort-based evaluation: Teaching children to evaluate their work based on effort and improvement rather than perfect outcomes.

Flexible thinking: Helping children understand that most problems have multiple valid solutions rather than one correct approach.

Mistake tolerance: Modeling how to handle errors as learning opportunities rather than failures that need prevention.

Process enjoyment: Encouraging children to find satisfaction in activities themselves rather than only in optimal results.

Personal value clarity: Helping children develop their own sense of what matters rather than automatically adopting others' priorities.

Relationship modeling:

Children learn relationship skills by watching how their parents interact. In OCPD families, this means actively modeling:

Respectful disagreement: Showing children how to maintain different approaches while still caring for each other.

Boundary respect: Demonstrating that people can have autonomy while still being part of a loving family.

Appreciation for differences: Celebrating various family members' different strengths and approaches rather than trying to optimize everyone into similarity.

Conflict resolution: Showing children how to address problems through collaboration rather than debate about whose way is superior.

Emotional validation: Modeling how to acknowledge and respect feelings even when they don't align with logical analysis.

The goal isn't to eliminate all standards or structure from children's lives. OCPD parents often provide valuable lessons about responsibility, planning, and excellence. The goal is ensuring that children learn these lessons without developing anxiety, perfectionism, or loss of confidence in their own judgment.

Practical approaches to shield children while maintaining family stability

Protecting children from harmful perfectionist pressure while preserving family relationships requires ongoing attention, flexibility, and commitment to both children's well-being and family cohesion.

The strategies in this chapter work together to create an environment where children can benefit from the OCPD parent's strengths while being protected from impossible standards. They help children develop resilience, maintain self-esteem, and learn healthy relationship skills that will serve them throughout their lives.

Most importantly, these approaches recognize that children's developmental needs must take priority over adult perfectionist preferences. While OCPD parents have legitimate needs for order and control, children's needs for exploration, mistake-making, and age-appropriate autonomy are equally important and must be protected.

This balance is challenging but achievable with consistent effort, clear communication, and professional support when needed. The goal is raising children who can appreciate excellence while accepting good enough, who can value different approaches while maintaining their own preferences, and who can navigate perfectionist pressure without losing their sense of self-worth and competence.

Your children deserve to feel confident, capable, and valued for who they are rather than how perfectly they perform. Protecting them from impossible standards while maintaining family stability is one of the most important investments you can make in their future well-being and relationship success.

Chapter 8: Getting your resistant partner into treatment

Michael had been researching therapists for three weeks, carefully reviewing credentials, treatment approaches, and client reviews. He'd found several excellent candidates who specialized in personality disorders and had experience with OCPD. But every time he tried to bring up the topic with his wife Jennifer, the conversation went nowhere.

"I think we could benefit from some relationship counseling," he'd say carefully.

"Why?" Jennifer would respond, genuinely puzzled. "What problems do you think we have that we can't solve ourselves?"

When Michael mentioned that her perfectionism created stress in their relationship, Jennifer looked confused. "I just want things done well. That's not perfectionism—that's having standards."

When he suggested that her need to control household decisions was causing conflict, she replied, "Someone has to make sure things get handled properly. If you want to take over more responsibilities, I'm happy to let you."

Jennifer wasn't being defensive or dismissive. She genuinely couldn't see any problems with her approach to their relationship that would require professional help. From her perspective, she was the responsible partner who maintained their household, planned efficiently, and tried to help Michael make better decisions. If there were problems in their relationship, they must stem from his resistance to obviously beneficial suggestions.

This is the central challenge of getting OCPD partners into treatment: **they don't experience their symptoms as problems.** Unlike depression (which feels terrible) or anxiety (which creates obvious distress), OCPD symptoms feel like solutions to other people's lack of care and attention to detail.

But here's what Michael eventually discovered: OCPD partners can be motivated to seek treatment, but only when the conversation appeals to their existing values of optimization, improvement, and achieving better outcomes. The key is framing therapy not as fixing problems they don't see, but as enhancing performance they already care about.

Why OCPD individuals resist therapy and how to overcome it

Understanding the specific reasons OCPD individuals avoid treatment is crucial for developing approaches that actually motivate them to seek help. Their resistance isn't stubbornness or denial—it's a logical response based on how their condition affects their thinking.

They genuinely don't see their behavior as problematic. Research shows that people with OCPD have significantly lower insight into their condition compared to other personality disorders (Pinto et al., 2014). They experience their rigid standards and controlling behaviors as appropriate responses to an inefficient, careless world. Seeking therapy for behavior that feels justified and helpful doesn't make logical sense to them.

They fear therapy will lower their standards. OCPD individuals often worry that treatment will make them less conscientious, organized, or achievement-oriented. They may have built their identity around being the responsible, thorough person who maintains high standards. The idea of changing these traits feels like becoming a lesser version of themselves.

They view emotional problems as efficiency issues. When OCPD individuals experience relationship conflicts or stress, they typically frame these as problems with communication efficiency, task

120

coordination, or decision-making processes rather than emotional or psychological issues requiring therapy. They're more likely to suggest better systems or clearer agreements than professional counseling.

They prefer self-reliance over outside help. The need to control outcomes extends to problem-solving approaches. OCPD individuals often believe they can research and implement solutions more effectively than relying on outside professionals. They may spend considerable time reading self-help books or developing their own improvement strategies rather than seeking therapy.

They're skeptical of therapeutic approaches that seem unstructured. Talk therapy can feel inefficient and imprecise to people who prefer clear goals, measurable outcomes, and systematic approaches to problem-solving. They may view therapy as too subjective or emotion-focused to produce reliable results.

Overcoming resistance requires strategic reframing:

Focus on performance enhancement rather than problem-fixing. Instead of presenting therapy as treatment for OCPD symptoms, position it as optimization of relationship functioning, communication efficiency, or stress management systems.

Emphasize measurable outcomes. Discuss therapy in terms of specific, observable improvements—better conflict resolution, more efficient household management, improved work-life balance, or enhanced family harmony.

Present research evidence. OCPD individuals respond well to data-driven arguments. Share statistics about therapy effectiveness, research on relationship improvement, or studies showing how certain approaches produce better outcomes.

Frame therapy as skill development. Position counseling as learning advanced techniques for communication, conflict resolution, stress management, or relationship optimization rather than fixing personality problems.

Address their expertise concerns. Acknowledge their competence in many areas while suggesting that relationship skills, like any other expertise, benefit from professional training and practice.

The Optimization Frame: Presenting therapy as performance enhancement

The most effective approach for motivating OCPD individuals toward treatment is presenting therapy as an opportunity to optimize areas of their lives that aren't currently performing at peak efficiency. This frame appeals to their natural drive for improvement while avoiding the stigma they associate with needing "help" for problems.

Relationship optimization framing:

"I've been thinking about how we could optimize our relationship functioning. We're both intelligent, capable people, but we seem to run into recurring inefficiencies in our communication and decision-making processes. I'd like to explore whether a relationship consultant could help us develop better systems for collaboration."

"We put effort into optimizing our finances, our home systems, and our career development. It seems logical to invest similar energy in optimizing our relationship performance. A couples therapist is essentially a relationship efficiency expert."

"I notice we spend significant time and energy on conflicts that don't seem to produce better outcomes for either of us. I'm wondering if there are more efficient approaches to handling disagreements that we could learn from a professional."

Stress management optimization:

"I can see that you experience frustration when things aren't done optimally. That stress doesn't seem to be producing the changes you want, so it's not an efficient use of your energy. Maybe there are better strategies for managing situations where you can't control the outcomes."

"You work really hard to maintain high standards, and I admire your dedication. I'm wondering if there are techniques for managing the stress that comes with caring so much about quality outcomes."

"It seems like you carry a lot of responsibility for ensuring things go well. That's admirable, but it also seems exhausting. Maybe a professional could suggest some strategies for managing that load more efficiently."

Communication skill development:

"I think we could both benefit from advanced communication training. We're both smart people, but we seem to have different communication styles that sometimes create inefficiency in our discussions."

"I've been reading about communication techniques that help people with different approaches work together more effectively. It might be worth consulting with someone who specializes in teaching these skills."

"I notice that when we disagree about methods or approaches, our discussions don't always lead to satisfactory resolutions for both of us. There might be better techniques we could learn for handling these situations."

Family system optimization:

"I want our family to function at its best possible level. That probably requires some advanced skills in areas like conflict resolution, stress management, and collaboration that we might not have learned naturally."

"We both want our children to develop good habits and standards. There might be more effective approaches to teaching these values without creating stress or resistance."

"I think we could be more efficient in how we handle household management and parenting responsibilities. A family systems consultant might have strategies we haven't considered."

The key elements of effective optimization framing:

Use business or technical language rather than therapy terminology. Words like "consultant," "efficiency," "optimization," "systems," and "performance" feel more comfortable than "counselor," "healing," "feelings," or "problems."

Focus on desired outcomes rather than current difficulties. Emphasize what you want to achieve rather than what's wrong with the current situation.

Acknowledge their competence while suggesting that even experts benefit from additional training and consultation in areas outside their primary expertise.

Present it as investment in important outcomes rather than fixing broken things. Frame therapy as optimization of already-functional systems rather than repair of damaged relationships.

Emphasize evidence-based approaches that appeal to their preference for research-supported methods rather than subjective or emotion-based interventions.

Scripts for the treatment conversation using five different approaches

Different OCPD individuals respond to different motivational approaches depending on their specific concerns, values, and relationship dynamics. Having multiple conversation strategies increases your chances of finding an approach that resonates with your particular partner.

Approach 1: The Research and Development Frame

"I've been researching ways to improve relationship satisfaction and found some interesting studies on couples therapy effectiveness. The research shows that couples who work with professionals achieve better outcomes than those who try to solve problems on their own. Given how much we both value evidence-based approaches, it seems worth investigating."

If they express skepticism: "I had the same initial reaction, but the data is pretty compelling. Studies show measurable improvements in communication efficiency, conflict resolution, and overall relationship satisfaction. The therapists who get the best results use structured, goal-oriented approaches rather than just talking about feelings."

If they say you can solve problems yourselves: "I agree that we're both capable problem-solvers. But even experts consult with other professionals to optimize their performance. Athletes have coaches, business leaders have consultants, and couples can benefit from relationship specialists who have expertise in areas we haven't studied extensively."

Approach 2: The Systems Improvement Frame

"I've noticed that we have some recurring patterns in our household management and communication that don't seem to be producing optimal outcomes. We're both smart people, but we might benefit from an outside perspective on how to improve our systems."

If they ask what problems you mean: "Not problems exactly, but inefficiencies. We spend time on disagreements that don't lead to better solutions, and sometimes our different approaches create friction instead of leveraging our different strengths. A systems consultant might help us design better processes."

If they suggest you can fix it yourselves: "Absolutely, and we've made improvements on our own. But most complex systems benefit from professional analysis at some point. We wouldn't try to optimize our financial portfolio without expert advice, so why not apply the same logic to optimizing our relationship system?"

Approach 3: The Stress Management Frame

"I can see how much energy you put into maintaining standards and ensuring things go well. That level of responsibility can be stressful, and I'm wondering if there are techniques for managing that stress more efficiently so it doesn't take such a toll on you."

If they deny being stressed: "Maybe stress isn't the right word. I'm talking about the mental energy you expend when things aren't done optimally. That energy is valuable, and there might be ways to channel it more effectively so you get better results with less effort."

If they say stress is normal: "I agree that caring about outcomes creates some pressure. But if there are strategies that help you achieve the same high standards with less frustration and anxiety, wouldn't that be worth exploring? It's like finding more efficient ways to accomplish any goal."

Approach 4: The Professional Development Frame

"I've been thinking about areas where we could both develop better skills. We invest in professional development for our careers, and it seems logical to invest in developing relationship and family management skills too."

If they question the need for skill development: "We're both competent in many areas, but relationship management involves some specialized skills that aren't taught in school or work settings. Communication techniques, conflict resolution, stress management—these are learnable skills that most people could improve with proper training."

If they prefer to learn on their own: "Self-directed learning is great, and we've both done a lot of that. But some skills are easier to develop with guided practice and feedback from someone who specializes in teaching them. It's like the difference between reading about a skill and having a qualified instructor help you refine your technique."

Approach 5: The Investment in Outcomes Frame

"Our relationship is one of our most important assets, and like any valuable asset, it probably benefits from professional maintenance and optimization. I'd like to invest in making sure we're getting the best possible outcomes from our partnership."

If they question the investment: "We spend money on maintaining our home, our cars, and our health because we want them to function optimally. Our relationship affects every other aspect of our lives, so investing in its performance seems like sound resource allocation."

If they worry about cost: "I've researched the costs, and relationship therapy is actually quite cost-effective compared to the expenses associated with relationship problems—lost productivity, health impacts from stress, potential impacts on our family. Prevention and optimization are usually much cheaper than dealing with problems after they develop."

Follow-up strategies for all approaches:

If they agree to consider it: "Great. I can research therapists who use evidence-based, structured approaches and specialize in helping couples optimize their relationships. Would you prefer someone with specific credentials or treatment methods?"

If they want to think about it: "That makes sense. Take whatever time you need to consider it. I can put together some research on different approaches and effectiveness rates if that would be helpful for your decision-making process."

If they suggest alternatives: "I'm open to trying other approaches first if you prefer. What timeframe should we set for evaluating whether alternative strategies are producing the improvements we want?"

What works: CBT, SSRIs, and Emotionally Focused Therapy

Understanding which treatments are most effective for OCPD can help you guide the conversation toward approaches that are more likely to produce positive outcomes. Research shows that certain therapeutic modalities and medications are particularly beneficial for OCPD individuals and their relationships.

Cognitive Behavioral Therapy remains the gold standard for OCPD treatment, with research demonstrating significant improvements in flexibility, perfectionism, and relationship satisfaction (Barber et al., 2007). CBT appeals to OCPD individuals because it's structured, goal-oriented, and focuses on changing specific behaviors rather than exploring deep emotional issues.

CBT for OCPD typically includes:

Cognitive restructuring that helps individuals recognize rigid thinking patterns and develop more flexible approaches to problems. This might involve identifying "should" statements, all-or-nothing thinking, and catastrophic predictions about suboptimal outcomes.

Behavioral experiments that test the consequences of doing things differently or accepting "good enough" outcomes. These experiments provide concrete evidence about whether perfectionist standards are truly necessary for acceptable results.

Exposure exercises that gradually increase tolerance for inefficiency, mess, and suboptimal outcomes in low-stakes situations. This helps reduce the anxiety that drives controlling behaviors.

Communication skills training that teaches more effective ways to express preferences and handle disagreements without becoming rigid or controlling.

Stress management techniques that help individuals cope with the anxiety they experience when things aren't done their preferred way.

When discussing CBT with your partner, emphasize its practical, skills-based approach: "CBT focuses on learning specific techniques for managing stress and improving communication rather than talking about childhood experiences or deep emotional issues. It's like technical training for relationship and stress management skills."

SSRI medications have shown significant effectiveness for OCPD symptoms, particularly the anxiety and depression that often accompany the condition (Ansell et al., 2010). While medications don't eliminate OCPD traits, they can reduce the intensity of perfectionist anxiety and make individuals more flexible in their thinking.

SSRIs that have shown benefits for OCPD include:

Fluoxetine (Prozac) has the most research support for OCPD symptoms and is often the first medication tried.

Sertraline (Zoloft) has shown effectiveness for perfectionist anxiety and rigid thinking patterns.

Paroxetine (Paxil) may be particularly helpful for individuals with significant anxiety about making mistakes or accepting suboptimal outcomes.

Citalopram (Celexa) has shown benefits for mood symptoms and interpersonal difficulties associated with OCPD.

When discussing medication options, frame them in terms of optimization rather than treatment for mental illness: "These medications help optimize brain chemistry to reduce the stress and anxiety that comes with caring deeply about outcomes. They don't change your personality or standards—they just make it easier to manage the emotional intensity that comes with perfectionism."

Emotionally Focused Therapy has shown promise for couples where one partner has OCPD (Johnson, 2019). EFT focuses on improving emotional connection and changing negative interaction cycles rather than trying to change individual personality traits.

EFT can be particularly effective for OCPD relationships because:

It doesn't require the OCPD partner to give up their standards but helps both partners understand how rigid standards affect emotional connection.

It focuses on interaction patterns rather than individual pathology, which feels less threatening to OCPD individuals.

It provides structured steps for improving communication and intimacy, which appeals to OCPD individuals' preference for systematic approaches.

It helps non-OCPD partners develop better responses to perfectionist pressure while helping OCPD partners understand the emotional impact of their behavior.

It addresses underlying attachment needs that may be driving controlling behaviors, offering alternative ways to feel secure in relationships.

When suggesting EFT, emphasize its focus on relationship systems: "Emotionally Focused Therapy helps couples understand their interaction patterns and develop more effective ways of connecting. It's not about changing who you are—it's about improving how you work together as a team."

Combination approaches often work best for OCPD individuals and their relationships. Many people benefit from individual CBT to address personal perfectionism and anxiety, medication to reduce symptom intensity, and couples therapy to improve relationship dynamics.

The treatment sequence might involve:

Starting with individual therapy to help the OCPD partner develop insight and skills before attempting couples work.

Adding medication if anxiety, depression, or rigid thinking are significantly impairing functioning.

Moving to couples therapy once the OCPD partner has developed some awareness of their patterns and is motivated to work on relationship improvement.

Ongoing maintenance through periodic check-ins or booster sessions to maintain progress and address new challenges.

Finding OCPD-informed therapists and questions to ask

Not all therapists have experience with OCPD, and working with someone who doesn't understand the condition can actually make things worse. OCPD individuals may feel misunderstood or unfairly pathologized by therapists who don't recognize the genuine benefits of their conscientious approach to life.

Essential qualifications to look for:

Experience with personality disorders is crucial, as OCPD requires different approaches than anxiety or depression treatment. Look for therapists who specifically mention personality disorders in their areas of expertise.

CBT training and experience ensures the therapist can provide the structured, goal-oriented treatment that works best for OCPD individuals.

Couples therapy expertise is important if you plan to work on relationship issues together. Look for training in EFT, Gottman Method, or other evidence-based couples approaches.

Understanding of high-functioning individuals helps ensure the therapist won't pathologize your partner's achievements and standards while still addressing problematic patterns.

Collaborative treatment approach that involves both partners in goal-setting and treatment planning rather than imposing external definitions of what needs to change.

Questions to ask potential therapists:

About OCPD experience: "How many clients with OCPD or obsessive-compulsive personality traits have you worked with?" "What approaches do you find most effective for helping OCPD individuals?" "How do you help clients maintain their strengths while addressing problematic patterns?" "What does treatment typically look like for someone with OCPD?"

About treatment approach: "Do you use structured, goal-oriented therapy approaches?" "How do you help clients who don't see their perfectionism as problematic?" "What role does medication play in your treatment of OCPD?" "How do you handle resistance to change in highly conscientious individuals?"

About couples work: "Do you work with couples where one partner has OCPD?" "How do you help non-OCPD partners cope with perfectionist pressure?" "What does couples therapy look like when perfectionism is creating relationship stress?" "How do you balance individual change with relationship improvement?"

About practical concerns: "What are your typical session frequency and treatment duration for OCPD?" "Do you provide homework or between-session assignments?" "How do you measure treatment progress?" "What should we expect in terms of timeline for seeing improvements?"

Red flags to avoid:

Therapists who immediately suggest personality change rather than symptom management and skill development.

Professionals who pathologize conscientiousness without recognizing its benefits and adaptive aspects.

Counselors who focus primarily on insight without providing concrete skills and strategies.

Therapists who can't explain their treatment approach in concrete, measurable terms.

Professionals who seem intimidated by high-functioning, analytical clients.

Online directories and referral sources:

Psychology Today allows you to filter by specialty areas including personality disorders, CBT, and couples therapy.

International OCD Foundation maintains referral lists for therapists experienced with obsessive-compulsive spectrum disorders.

American Association for Marriage and Family Therapy provides referrals for couples therapists with specific expertise areas.

Your primary care physician may be able to provide referrals to mental health professionals familiar with OCPD.

Employee assistance programs through work may offer referrals to therapists with experience treating high-functioning professionals.

When calling potential therapists, briefly explain your situation: "I'm looking for a therapist who has experience with OCPD or obsessive-compulsive personality traits. My partner is highly conscientious and detail-oriented, which has many benefits, but it's also creating some stress in our relationship. I'm hoping to find someone who can help us work on relationship dynamics while respecting my partner's strengths."

Preparing for resistance and building motivation over time

Even with perfect framing and excellent therapist selection, many OCPD individuals need time to warm up to the idea of treatment. Building motivation is often a gradual process rather than a single conversation.

Stages of readiness to expect:

Initial resistance where your partner sees no need for outside help and may feel criticized by the suggestion that anything needs improvement.

Intellectual curiosity where they begin researching therapy approaches, reading about relationship improvement, or asking questions about what treatment involves.

Conditional willingness where they agree to try therapy with specific conditions—time limits, particular approaches, or trial periods.

Active engagement where they participate in treatment and begin implementing suggestions and strategies.

Investment in the process where they see benefits and become motivated to continue working on improvement.

Building motivation strategies:

Plant seeds gradually rather than pushing for immediate decisions. Mention articles you've read, share research you've found, or discuss other couples who've benefited from therapy.

Address specific concerns they raise about therapy rather than giving generic reassurances. If they worry about time investment, research efficient therapy approaches. If they fear judgment, find therapists who work with high-functioning professionals.

Offer control over the process. Let them research therapists, choose the approach, or set the timeline. OCPD individuals are more likely to engage when they feel they're directing their own improvement process.

Start with less threatening options. They might be more willing to read self-help books, attend workshops, or try online resources before committing to individual therapy.

Connect therapy to their existing goals. Frame treatment as supporting their career success, parenting effectiveness, or other outcomes they already care about.

Managing your own frustration during this process is crucial for maintaining the long-term perspective needed to motivate change:

Accept that this is a marathon, not a sprint. OCPD individuals often take months or even years to move from initial resistance to active engagement in treatment.

Focus on small progress rather than expecting dramatic shifts in attitude. Celebrate when they show curiosity, ask questions, or express any openness to the idea.

Maintain your own boundaries about what you need for your mental health while giving them time to consider treatment options.

Get support for yourself through individual therapy, support groups, or trusted friends who understand the challenges you're facing.

Don't make treatment a ultimatum unless you're genuinely prepared to follow through on consequences. Empty threats damage trust and reduce your credibility for future conversations.

What to do if they absolutely refuse treatment

Some OCPD individuals will never voluntarily engage in treatment, regardless of how well you frame the conversation or how much evidence you provide. In these cases, you have several options for managing your situation while protecting your own well-being.

Focus on your own growth and support:

Individual therapy can provide you with strategies for managing OCPD relationship dynamics, maintaining your mental health, and making decisions about your future.

Support groups for partners of people with personality disorders offer validation, practical advice, and connection with others facing similar challenges.

Relationship education through books, workshops, or online resources can help you develop better responses to perfectionist pressure even without your partner's participation.

Personal boundaries and self-care become even more important when your partner isn't working on their contribution to relationship problems.

Set clear expectations about change:

Communicate your needs clearly about what has to change for the relationship to remain sustainable for you, even if your partner isn't willing to seek professional help.

Establish consequences for behavior that significantly impacts your mental health, and follow through consistently.

Build your support network and maintain connections outside your relationship that provide perspective and emotional support.

Plan for various outcomes including the possibility that your partner's unwillingness to work on the relationship may require you to make difficult decisions about your future.

Consider couples therapy without them:

Some therapists will work with individuals to address relationship dynamics even when their partner won't participate. This can help you develop better strategies for managing OCPD behavior and making decisions about your relationship.

Try alternative approaches:

Self-help resources specifically designed for OCPD relationships can provide strategies and insights even without professional guidance.

Relationship workshops or retreats might feel less threatening than therapy to some OCPD individuals.

Online therapy platforms may seem more efficient and convenient than traditional counseling.

Pastoral counseling or spiritual guidance might appeal to OCPD individuals who are uncomfortable with mental health treatment.

The most important thing to understand is that you cannot force someone into therapy, and you cannot fix your relationship alone. Your partner's willingness to work on their contribution to relationship problems is ultimately their choice. Your job is to take care of yourself, set appropriate boundaries, and make informed decisions about what you can and cannot accept in your relationship.

Building hope while maintaining realistic expectations

The good news is that many OCPD individuals do eventually become motivated to seek treatment, especially when they begin to see how their patterns affect their relationships, careers, or overall life satisfaction. The process often takes longer than partners hope, but change is possible.

What you can realistically expect from treatment:

OCPD individuals can learn to recognize their rigid thinking patterns and develop more flexibility in their responses. They can reduce the intensity of their perfectionist anxiety and become more tolerant of suboptimal outcomes. They can improve their communication skills and develop better awareness of how their behavior affects others.

What's unlikely to change completely:

Your partner will probably always prefer order, structure, and high standards. They'll likely continue to notice inefficiencies and suboptimal approaches. Their natural inclination will be toward thorough planning and systematic approaches to tasks and decisions.

The goal of treatment isn't to eliminate OCPD traits entirely—it's to help your partner manage these traits in ways that don't create distress for themselves or their relationships. Many people with OCPD learn to channel their conscientiousness in positive directions while developing tolerance for situations they can't control.

Treatment works best when both partners are committed to improvement and when the OCPD individual is genuinely motivated to develop more flexibility. With the right combination of therapy, possibly medication, and consistent effort, many couples do find ways to create more balanced, satisfying relationships while honoring both partners' needs and strengths.

Your patience and strategic approach to motivating treatment can make a significant difference in whether your partner becomes willing to work on these issues. The conversation about therapy may not succeed the first time, or even the fifth time, but consistent, respectful encouragement often does eventually lead to openness to getting help.

Strategic approaches that actually motivate treatment-seeking

The strategies in this chapter work because they respect your partner's OCPD thinking while creating motivation for change. They frame therapy as optimization rather than problem-solving, appeal to their values of efficiency and improvement, and provide them with control over the treatment process.

Most importantly, these approaches acknowledge that change takes time and that building motivation is often more effective than creating ultimatums. OCPD individuals can and do change, but they need to feel that treatment aligns with their goals and values rather than contradicting their fundamental approach to life.

Your persistence, patience, and strategic thinking about how to present treatment options can be the difference between ongoing relationship struggle and genuine improvement. The effort you put into understanding their perspective and framing treatment appropriately is an investment in both your partner's well-being and your relationship's future.

Chapter 9: The decision framework

Should you stay or should you go?

Sarah sat at her kitchen table at 2 AM, staring at a list she'd been creating for weeks. On one side: "Reasons to Stay." On the other: "Reasons to Leave." The middle of the page remained blank—a space for the decision she couldn't seem to make.

Reasons to Stay:

- He's not abusive or cruel

- He genuinely cares and tries to help

- We have good financial stability

- He's an excellent father in many ways

- His standards have improved some aspects of our life

- I made a commitment for better or worse

Reasons to Leave:

- I feel like I'm disappearing

- Nothing I do feels good enough

- I'm exhausted from walking on eggshells

- The kids are developing anxiety about mistakes

- I can't remember who I was before his standards

- I don't see this getting significantly better

Both lists felt true. Both lists felt incomplete. The rational part of Sarah's brain said that relationships require compromise and that her husband Mark wasn't intentionally harmful. The emotional part of her brain screamed that she was suffocating under the weight of constant optimization and correction.

Sarah's dilemma reflects the complexity of OCPD relationships. These aren't clear-cut situations with obvious answers. They're nuanced, challenging dynamics where genuine love and care coexist with patterns that can be slowly destructive to one partner's sense of self.

Making the decision to stay or leave requires a framework that goes beyond simple lists of pros and cons. It requires honest assessment of what's actually changeable, what you can realistically accept long-term, and what your life might look like under different scenarios.

This chapter provides tools for making one of the most important decisions of your life with clarity, objectivity, and full awareness of the complex factors involved.

The Stay/Leave Assessment Matrix

Traditional decision-making approaches often fail with OCPD relationships because they don't account for the unique factors these partnerships involve. The Stay/Leave Assessment Matrix evaluates your situation across multiple dimensions that specifically matter in perfectionist relationships.

Dimension 1: Partner's insight and willingness to change

High insight/High willingness (Stay-favorable): Your partner recognizes that their standards create stress for you and the family. They're willing to work on flexibility and compromise. They may not see their behavior as a disorder, but they acknowledge its impact on others and want to improve.

Moderate insight/Moderate willingness (Neutral): Your partner sometimes recognizes their rigidity but often justifies it as necessary.

They're willing to make minor adjustments but resistant to major changes in their approach. They may agree to therapy or compromises during conflicts but revert to old patterns during stress.

Low insight/Low willingness (Leave-favorable): Your partner sees no problems with their standards and believes others should adapt. They view suggestions for change as unreasonable requests to lower quality or accept inferior outcomes. They may become angry or defensive when their methods are questioned.

Dimension 2: Impact on your mental health

Minimal impact (Stay-favorable): You feel challenged sometimes but maintain confidence in your abilities and judgment. You have strategies for managing perfectionist pressure and don't feel like you're losing yourself. Your self-esteem remains intact despite occasional conflicts.

Moderate impact (Neutral): You experience periods of self-doubt and frustration but can usually recover your equilibrium. You've developed some coping strategies but still struggle with feeling adequate. Your mental health has ups and downs related to relationship stress.

Severe impact (Leave-favorable): You frequently question your competence and judgment. You experience anxiety, depression, or other mental health symptoms related to relationship dynamics. You feel like you're losing your sense of self or becoming someone you don't recognize.

Dimension 3: Children's wellbeing

Positive/protected (Stay-favorable): Children benefit from structure and high standards while being protected from impossible expectations. They show normal confidence, creativity, and willingness to take risks. Both parents support their development appropriately.

Mixed impact (Neutral): Children receive some benefits from high standards but also experience stress from perfectionist pressure. They show some signs of anxiety or perfectionism but maintain overall emotional health. Interventions are helping protect them from negative impacts.

Negative impact (Leave-favorable): Children show signs of anxiety, perfectionism, or fear of making mistakes. They're becoming overly cautious or developing low self-esteem. The perfectionist environment is significantly affecting their emotional development or academic confidence.

Dimension 4: Relationship trajectory

Improving (Stay-favorable): Conflicts are decreasing in frequency and intensity. Both partners are developing better communication and compromise skills. Small but consistent improvements suggest continued progress is possible.

Stable (Neutral): The relationship maintains a consistent pattern with both positive and challenging elements. Problems aren't getting worse, but significant improvement seems unlikely without major changes.

Deteriorating (Leave-favorable): Conflicts are increasing or becoming more intense. Resentment is building on both sides. Previous improvements aren't being maintained, and the overall dynamic seems to be getting worse over time.

Dimension 5: Support systems and resources

Strong support (Stay-favorable): You have access to therapy, supportive friends and family, and resources for managing relationship stress. Your partner is willing to work with professionals and accepts outside input about relationship dynamics.

Moderate support (Neutral): You have some support but may lack comprehensive resources or professional guidance. Your partner has mixed reactions to outside involvement but isn't completely resistant to help.

Limited support (Leave-favorable): You feel isolated and lack access to professional help or supportive relationships. Your partner resists outside involvement and may discourage you from seeking support or maintaining connections that provide perspective.

Matrix scoring:

Rate your relationship on each dimension from 1 (strongly leave-favorable) to 5 (strongly stay-favorable):

- Partner insight/willingness: ____

- Mental health impact: ____

- Children's wellbeing: ____

- Relationship trajectory: ____

- Support/resources: ____

Total score: ____/25

Score interpretation:

- 20-25: Relationship has strong potential for positive outcomes with continued effort

- 15-19: Mixed indicators suggest relationship could work with significant improvements

- 10-14: Serious concerns require major changes for relationship sustainability

- 5-9: Multiple severe issues suggest leaving may be the healthier choice

This matrix provides objective framework, but the final decision must also consider your personal values, circumstances, and intuitive sense of what's right for your situation.

Financial planning for potential separation

One of the most practical barriers to leaving OCPD relationships is financial concerns. OCPD partners are often high earners and financial managers, which can create economic dependence that complicates decision-making. Planning financially for potential separation provides you with options and reduces the fear that keeps many people in unsustainable relationships.

Immediate financial assessment:

Personal income and assets: Document your current earning capacity, savings, investments, and any assets in your name only. This gives you baseline information about your independent financial position.

Joint assets and debts: Create comprehensive list of all shared financial obligations and assets, including bank accounts, retirement funds, real estate, vehicles, and debts. Understand what would be subject to division in separation.

Monthly expenses: Track your actual spending to understand what your independent household budget would need to cover. Include housing, utilities, food, transportation, insurance, and child-related expenses.

Earning potential: Assess your ability to increase income through career advancement, additional education, or returning to work if you've been out of the workforce. Consider what steps would be needed to achieve financial independence.

Hidden financial vulnerabilities: OCPD partners often manage finances completely, leaving their partners unaware of the full financial picture. Ensure you understand all accounts, investments, insurance policies, and financial obligations.

Building financial independence:

Separate savings account: Start saving money in an account your partner doesn't control or monitor. Even small amounts build up over time and provide security for emergencies or transition expenses.

Credit establishment: If you don't have credit in your own name, work on establishing credit history through a secured credit card or small loan. Good credit is essential for renting apartments, getting utilities, or making other independent financial arrangements.

Career development: Invest in skills, education, or networking that would improve your earning potential if you needed to support yourself. This might include updating certifications, taking classes, or reconnecting with professional contacts.

Legal consultation: Meet with a family law attorney to understand your rights regarding asset division, spousal support, and child custody. Many attorneys offer free initial consultations or sliding-scale fees.

Support system development: Build relationships with people who could provide temporary housing, emotional support, or practical assistance if you needed to leave quickly. This reduces dependence on financial resources alone.

Separation cost planning:

Housing deposits and moving expenses: First month's rent, security deposits, utility connections, and moving costs can easily total several thousand dollars. Plan for these upfront expenses.

Legal fees: Attorney fees for divorce or separation agreements typically range from a few thousand to tens of thousands of dollars, depending on complexity and cooperation level.

Therapy and counseling: Individual therapy for yourself and possibly your children requires budgeting for ongoing mental health support during transition.

Childcare and support: If you'll have primary custody, budget for increased childcare costs, school expenses, and child support calculations.

Lifestyle adjustments: Your post-separation standard of living will likely be different. Plan for changes in housing, transportation, entertainment, and other expenses.

Long-term financial planning:

Retirement considerations: Understand how separation would affect retirement savings and long-term financial security. Some retirement accounts require special handling in divorce proceedings.

Insurance coverage: Plan for health, life, and disability insurance that isn't dependent on your partner's employer coverage.

Education funding: If you have children, consider how college savings and educational expenses would be handled after separation.

Emergency fund building: Work toward having 3-6 months of living expenses saved for unexpected costs or income interruptions.

Financial planning resources:

Financial advisors can help you understand your current situation and develop strategies for independence. Look for fee-only advisors who don't sell products.

Credit counseling services offer free or low-cost assistance with budgeting, debt management, and credit improvement.

Legal aid organizations provide low-cost legal assistance for people with limited income who need help with family law issues.

Women's resource centers often offer financial planning workshops, career counseling, and practical support for people considering leaving relationships.

Online tools and calculators can help you estimate separation costs, understand asset division, and plan budgets for independent living.

The goal isn't necessarily to leave your relationship, but to have the financial security that allows you to make decisions based on what's best for your wellbeing rather than economic fear.

Trial separation as diagnostic tool

Sometimes the only way to truly understand whether your relationship is sustainable is to experience life apart from your partner's perfectionist pressure. Trial separations can provide valuable information about how both partners function independently and whether absence creates motivation for change.

When trial separation might be helpful:

You're uncertain about your feelings and can't tell whether you're unhappy because of changeable relationship dynamics or because of fundamental incompatibility.

Your partner lacks insight into how their behavior affects others and might develop awareness through experiencing the consequences of their actions.

You've lost touch with yourself and need space to rediscover your preferences, confidence, and decision-making ability without constant input.

Children are being affected by household tension, and temporary separation might provide them with relief while parents work on individual issues.

Previous attempts at change haven't worked and both partners need to understand what they're willing to do to preserve the relationship.

Structured trial separation planning:

Duration and goals: Agree on specific timeframe (typically 3-6 months) and what both partners hope to accomplish during the separation. Clear goals prevent the separation from becoming indefinite limbo.

Living arrangements: Decide who stays in the family home and where the other partner will live. Consider impact on children, finances, and both partners' comfort and stability.

Communication agreements: Establish rules about how much contact you'll have and what topics are appropriate to discuss. Some couples benefit from structured weekly check-ins, while others need more space.

Financial arrangements: Agree on how expenses will be handled during separation, including mortgage/rent, utilities, childcare, and individual living costs.

Child custody and parenting: Create clear schedule for when children are with each parent and how decisions about their care will be made during the separation period.

Therapy and support: Many couples benefit from individual therapy during separation to work on personal issues and couples therapy to process the experience.

What to evaluate during trial separation:

Your mental health and energy levels: Do you feel more relaxed, confident, and energetic without daily exposure to perfectionist pressure? Or do you feel lost and anxious without your partner's structure and guidance?

Decision-making confidence: Can you make daily decisions without anxiety or second-guessing? Do you trust your judgment more or less when you're not receiving constant input?

Relationship with children: If you have kids, do they seem more relaxed or more stressed during the separation? How do they adjust to different household standards?

Daily life management: Can you handle household tasks, finances, and daily responsibilities without your partner's systems and standards? Do you prefer more flexibility or do you miss the structure?

Social connections: Do you reconnect with friends and activities that you'd drifted away from? Do you feel more or less socially confident?

Future vision: Can you imagine being happy long-term in either scenario—with or without your partner? What would each path require from you?

Your partner's response: Do they use the separation as motivation to work on their rigidity and control issues? Do they develop insight into how their behavior affects relationships? Or do they blame you for being unreasonable?

Common outcomes of trial separations:

Renewed commitment with changes: Both partners gain perspective on what they need to change, develop better appreciation for each other, and return to relationship with new agreements and approaches.

Peaceful separation: Both partners realize they're happier apart and can work together to create amicable divorce or permanent separation that protects everyone's wellbeing.

Temporary relief followed by same patterns: The separation provides short-term relief, but when partners reunite, the same dynamics quickly reestablish themselves without lasting change.

Increased conflict: The separation creates more stress and anger, making it harder to work together on solutions or peaceful resolution.

Clarity about deal-breakers: The experience helps both partners understand what they absolutely cannot accept in relationships and whether those issues are changeable.

Trial separations aren't right for every situation, and they should be entered with careful planning and realistic expectations. They're tools for gaining information and perspective, not strategies for pressuring partners into change.

When leaving becomes necessary: Clear warning signs

While many OCPD relationships can improve with appropriate strategies and professional help, some situations become dangerous or unsustainable. Recognizing these warning signs can help you make decisions that protect your safety and wellbeing.

Mental health crisis indicators:

Severe depression or anxiety that's directly related to relationship dynamics and doesn't improve despite individual therapy and medication.

Suicidal thoughts or self-harm resulting from feelings of hopelessness about your relationship or life situation.

Complete loss of identity where you can't access your own preferences, values, or decision-making ability after extended exposure to control and criticism.

Panic attacks or physical symptoms triggered by your partner's criticism or perfectionist episodes.

Substance abuse as coping mechanism for relationship stress or to numb feelings of inadequacy and frustration.

Escalation patterns:

Physical intimidation or aggression during perfectionist episodes, even if your partner hasn't been physically violent in the past.

Emotional abuse disguised as help where criticism becomes personally attacking rather than focused on methods or outcomes.

Isolation from support systems where your partner actively discourages or prevents you from maintaining relationships that provide perspective.

Financial control that prevents you from accessing money, credit, or resources you need for independence.

Threats or ultimatums about relationship consequences if you don't comply with their standards or demands.

Children in danger:

Emotional abuse of children through impossible standards, harsh criticism, or punishment for normal childhood behavior.

Anxiety disorders developing in children related to perfectionist pressure and fear of making mistakes.

Academic or social problems resulting from children's anxiety about meeting parental expectations.

Physical symptoms in children such as headaches, stomachaches, or sleep problems related to household stress.

Developmental delays in independence, creativity, or social skills due to overcontrol and micromanagement.

Relationship deterioration:

Complete breakdown of communication where discussions always become arguments about methods and standards.

Escalating resentment on both sides that makes daily interaction difficult and unpleasant.

Loss of all intimacy and emotional connection due to the power dynamics created by perfectionist control.

Repeated failed attempts at improvement despite professional help, medication, and genuine effort from both partners.

Partner's unwillingness to acknowledge any problems or take responsibility for their contribution to relationship difficulties.

Safety planning for leaving:

Document concerning incidents including dates, details, and any evidence of escalating behavior that might be relevant in custody or legal proceedings.

Build financial resources and establish credit independently so you can support yourself and your children during transition.

Connect with professional support including therapists, attorneys, and domestic violence resources even if physical violence hasn't occurred.

Develop safety network of friends, family, or professional contacts who can provide assistance if you need to leave quickly.

Plan for children's needs including school arrangements, therapy, and maintaining stability during transition.

Understand legal rights regarding asset division, spousal support, and child custody before making any final decisions.

Emergency resources:

National Domestic Violence Hotline (1-800-799-7233) provides 24/7 support even for emotional abuse situations.

Local women's shelters often provide counseling, legal advocacy, and practical support for leaving relationships.

Family law attorneys can help you understand your rights and options before you make any decisions about leaving.

Mental health crisis services are available through hospitals, community mental health centers, and crisis hotlines.

Employee assistance programs through work may provide counseling, legal consultation, and other support services.

Leaving isn't failure, and staying isn't automatically success. The right decision depends on your specific situation, your partner's willingness to change, and your own wellbeing and safety.

Decision-making worksheet with weighted factors

Different factors matter more to different people depending on their values, circumstances, and life stage. This worksheet helps you identify which considerations are most important to you and evaluate your situation accordingly.

Step 1: Factor importance weighting

Rate how important each factor is to you personally on a scale of 1-10:

Your mental health and wellbeing: ___ **Children's emotional and developmental health:** ___ **Financial security and stability:** ___ **Partner's willingness to change and grow:** ___ **Quality of daily life and household peace:** ___ **Social connections and support systems:** ___ **Personal growth and self-actualization:** ___ **Commitment and marriage values:** ___ **Family stability and continuity:** ___ **Professional/career considerations:** ___

Step 2: Current situation assessment

Rate how well each factor is currently being met in your relationship on a scale of 1-10:

Your mental health and wellbeing: ___ **Children's emotional and developmental health:** ___ **Financial security and stability:** ___ **Partner's willingness to change and grow:** ___ **Quality of daily life and household peace:** ___ **Social connections and support systems:** ___ **Personal growth and self-actualization:** ___ **Commitment and marriage values:** ___ **Family stability and continuity:** ___ **Professional/career considerations:** ___

Step 3: Weighted calculation

For each factor, multiply importance rating by current satisfaction rating:

Mental health: ___ × ___ = ___

Children's health: ___ × ___ = ___

Financial security: ___ × ___ = ___

Partner's willingness: ___ × ___ = ___

Daily life quality: ___ × ___ = ___

Social connections: ___ × ___ = ___

Personal growth: ___ × ___ = ___

Commitment values: ___ × ___ = ___

Family stability: ___ × ___ = ___

Career considerations: ___ × ___ = ___

Total current relationship score: ___/1000

Step 4: Future scenarios evaluation

Scenario A: Staying with significant improvements Rate each factor assuming your partner makes substantial changes and you work together on relationship improvement:

Mental health: ___ **Children's health:** ___ **Financial security:** ___ **Partner's willingness:** ___ **Daily life quality:** ___ **Social connections:** ___ **Personal growth:** ___ **Commitment values:** ___ **Family stability:** ___ **Career considerations:** ___

Calculate weighted scores and total: ___/1000

Scenario B: Staying with minimal changes Rate each factor assuming your relationship continues with only minor improvements:

Calculate weighted scores and total: ___/1000

Scenario C: Amicable separation Rate each factor assuming you separate peacefully with good co-parenting and mutual respect:

Calculate weighted scores and total: ___/1000

Scenario D: Difficult separation Rate each factor assuming separation involves conflict, legal battles, and ongoing tension:

Calculate weighted scores and total: ___/1000

Step 5: Scenario likelihood assessment

Rate the probability of each scenario on a scale of 1-10:

Staying with significant improvements: ___ Staying with minimal changes: ___ Amicable separation: ___ Difficult separation: ___

Step 6: Decision framework questions

Which scenario scores highest when you multiply the weighted satisfaction score by the likelihood rating?

What factors are most important to you, and how well would they be met under different scenarios?

What changes would need to occur for your relationship to meet your weighted priority requirements?

What timeframe is reasonable for evaluating whether necessary changes are happening?

What support do you need to implement whichever decision you make?

Additional considerations:

Values alignment: Do your core values support working on the relationship or prioritize individual wellbeing and autonomy?

Energy and resources: Do you have the emotional, physical, and financial resources required for relationship improvement work?

Partner's trajectory: Is your partner moving toward greater insight and flexibility, or do they seem increasingly rigid and resistant?

Children's input: If age-appropriate, what do your children's needs and preferences suggest about the best path forward?

Professional guidance: What do therapists, counselors, or other professionals recommend based on their assessment of your situation?

Gut instinct: What does your intuition tell you about what's right for your life, separate from logical analysis?

This worksheet provides structure for decision-making, but the final choice must align with your personal values, circumstances, and sense of what will create the best outcomes for everyone involved.

Living with your decision once made

Whether you decide to stay and continue working on your relationship or to leave and rebuild your life independently, the decision-making process doesn't end when you choose a path. Both options require ongoing commitment, adjustment, and support to succeed.

If you decide to stay:

Commit fully to the improvement process rather than staying while mentally preparing to leave. Half-hearted effort rarely produces the changes needed for relationship success.

Maintain clear boundaries about what changes are necessary and what timeline is reasonable for seeing improvement.

Invest in ongoing support through individual therapy, couples counseling, or support groups to help navigate the ongoing challenges.

Regular progress assessment helps ensure you're making genuine progress rather than just adapting to unsustainable dynamics.

Preserve your individual identity and relationships outside the partnership so you don't lose yourself in the improvement process.

If you decide to leave:

Follow through with appropriate professional support including legal counsel, therapy, and practical assistance with transition logistics.

Focus on creating stability for yourself and your children rather than trying to change your partner's understanding of your decision.

Maintain respect and cooperation when possible, especially when children are involved, while protecting your own boundaries and wellbeing.

Build your independent life systematically rather than just reacting to the absence of your former relationship.

Process the grief and loss that comes with ending a significant relationship, even when leaving was the right decision.

Both paths require:

Self-compassion for the difficulty of the situation and recognition that there were no perfect solutions available.

Ongoing professional support to help you navigate whatever path you choose successfully.

Patience with the process of change and adjustment, which takes time regardless of which direction you go.

Focus on your children's needs and providing them with stability and support during whatever transition occurs.

Commitment to your own growth and mental health regardless of your relationship status.

The goal isn't to make a perfect decision—it's to make the best decision you can with the information available and then commit to making that decision work as well as possible for everyone involved.

Objective framework for life-changing decisions

The decision framework in this chapter provides structure for one of the most complex choices you may ever face. It acknowledges that OCPD relationships involve unique factors that traditional relationship advice doesn't address, while providing objective tools for evaluating your specific situation.

Most importantly, this framework recognizes that both staying and leaving can be valid choices depending on your circumstances, your partner's willingness to change, and your own values and priorities. There's no universal right answer—only the answer that's right for your specific situation and the people involved.

The tools in this chapter help you move beyond the emotional confusion that often accompanies these decisions and create a clear-eyed assessment of your options, their likely outcomes, and the resources you'll need to succeed regardless of which path you choose.

Your decision deserves careful consideration, professional support, and respect for the complexity of your situation. Whether you stay or leave, you deserve a life that supports your mental health, honors your values, and allows you to feel confident about the choice you've made.

Chapter 10: Success stories— relationships that turned around

Three years ago, Janet was sitting in her therapist's office, tissues in hand, describing a marriage that felt impossible to fix. Her husband Paul's need to optimize every aspect of their lives had created a household where she felt constantly evaluated and never quite adequate. Their teenage daughter had developed anxiety about making mistakes. Their son had stopped bringing friends home because Paul would reorganize their activities for "better outcomes."

"I love him," Janet told her therapist, "but I feel like I'm drowning in his improvements."

Last month, Janet and Paul celebrated their twentieth wedding anniversary with a trip that included both planned activities (Paul's preference) and spontaneous adventures (Janet's choice). Their daughter is thriving in college, confident and creative. Their son regularly hosts friends at home, where they enjoy the structure Paul provides while feeling accepted for their imperfect teenage approach to life.

The transformation didn't happen overnight, and it wasn't magic. It was the result of medication that helped Paul manage his anxiety about suboptimal outcomes, therapy that gave both partners new tools for communication and compromise, and consistent work from both people to create a relationship that honored their different needs.

Janet and Paul's story is one of several we'll explore in this chapter— real examples of OCPD relationships that found ways to balance perfectionism with flexibility, control with autonomy, and individual needs with partnership success. These stories don't promise easy solutions, but they demonstrate that change is possible when both partners are committed to improvement.

The medication breakthrough: How SSRIs changed everything

Rebecca had lived with David's perfectionism for twelve years before she understood that his behavior might have a medical component. She'd tried every relationship strategy she could find—better communication, clearer boundaries, couples therapy—but David's need to control household systems and correct her methods remained constant.

The turning point came during a routine physical when David mentioned to his doctor that he was having trouble sleeping because his mind kept cycling through all the inefficient ways people around him handled tasks. "It's like I can see the better solution, but I can't turn off thinking about it," he explained.

His physician suggested that this kind of repetitive, anxiety-driven thinking might benefit from medication and referred David to a psychiatrist who specialized in anxiety and obsessive-compulsive spectrum disorders.

The medication trial process:

David was initially resistant to the idea of psychiatric medication. "I don't have a mental illness," he told Rebecca. "I just care about doing things well." But his sleep disruption was affecting his work performance, and he was willing to try medication if it would help him manage the mental cycling that kept him awake.

The psychiatrist explained that SSRI medications can help reduce the anxiety and rigidity associated with perfectionist thinking patterns. "This won't change your personality or your ability to maintain high standards," she told David. "It should help you feel less distressed when things aren't done optimally and give you more choice about when to apply your standards."

David started on a low dose of sertraline (Zoloft) with careful monitoring for side effects and effectiveness. The changes were gradual but significant.

Month 1: David's sleep improved as his mind became less active at bedtime. He was still noticing inefficiencies around him, but the observations felt less urgent and compelling.

Month 2: Rebecca noticed that David was less likely to take over tasks she was working on. He would still make suggestions, but he could accept her declining to implement them without becoming frustrated or insistent.

Month 3: David began experimenting with accepting "good enough" outcomes in low-stakes situations. He let Rebecca load the dishwasher her way without reorganizing it, and was surprised to discover that the dishes got just as clean.

Month 6: The family's stress level decreased significantly as David became more flexible about methods and standards. He maintained his organizational systems and high standards in areas that mattered most to him while relaxing his expectations in areas that were less critical.

Long-term outcomes:

Two years later, David continues taking medication and describes it as "giving me choice about when to be perfectionist rather than feeling like I have to optimize everything." He's maintained his strengths—excellent planning, attention to detail, high-quality work—while developing tolerance for his family's different approaches.

Rebecca reports feeling like she has her husband back. "He's still David—organized, thorough, conscientious—but he's not driven by anxiety about imperfection anymore. He can enjoy our family's chaos without needing to fix it constantly."

Their teenage sons have noticed the change too. "Dad still helps us with homework and expects us to do our best," their older son explains, "but he doesn't freak out if we do things differently than he would. He's more fun to be around."

Key factors in medication success:

Proper diagnosis: Working with a psychiatrist who understood OCPD and could distinguish it from other conditions was crucial for selecting appropriate medication and dosage.

Gradual expectations: David and Rebecca didn't expect dramatic personality changes but looked for subtle improvements in flexibility and anxiety management.

Combination with therapy: David also worked with a cognitive-behavioral therapist to develop skills for managing perfectionist thinking and tolerating imperfection.

Family support: Rebecca and the children learned to appreciate David's improvements without expecting him to become a completely different person.

Long-term commitment: David views medication as a tool for managing a chronic condition rather than a temporary fix, which has helped maintain the improvements.

Realistic outcomes: The medication didn't eliminate David's perfectionism or high standards—it reduced the anxiety that made those standards feel urgent and non-negotiable.

Research supports David and Rebecca's experience. Studies show that SSRIs can be particularly effective for reducing the anxiety and rigidity associated with OCPD, especially when combined with cognitive-behavioral therapy (Ansell et al., 2010). The medications don't change personality but can reduce symptom intensity enough to allow for greater flexibility and choice in applying perfectionist standards.

The therapy success: Couple who found their way back

Mark and Jennifer had reached a breaking point after fifteen years of marriage. Mark's OCPD had created a household dynamic where Jennifer felt like she was failing at basic adult competence while Mark felt frustrated by her apparent resistance to obviously beneficial improvements.

Their relationship had developed a predictable cycle: Jennifer would attempt tasks using her natural approach, Mark would offer corrections or take over to ensure optimal results, Jennifer would feel criticized and inadequate, and both would become increasingly frustrated with each other.

"We were like two people speaking different languages," Jennifer recalls. "He thought he was being helpful, and I felt like nothing I did was ever good enough."

The therapy journey:

Mark and Jennifer found a couples therapist who specialized in relationships where one partner had perfectionist or obsessive-compulsive traits. Their therapist, Dr. Amanda Chen, used Emotionally Focused Therapy (EFT) combined with cognitive-behavioral techniques to help them understand their interaction patterns and develop new ways of connecting.

Phase 1: Pattern identification (Sessions 1-6)

Dr. Chen helped Mark and Jennifer map their negative cycle:

- Jennifer attempts task using her preferred method
- Mark experiences anxiety about suboptimal outcomes
- Mark offers corrections or improvements
- Jennifer feels criticized and inadequate
- Jennifer withdraws or becomes defensive
- Mark feels rejected and misunderstood

- Both partners become more entrenched in their positions

Understanding this cycle helped both partners recognize that their individual responses made sense but created a dynamic that left both people feeling unsuccessful and disconnected.

Phase 2: Emotional exploration (Sessions 7-12)

Dr. Chen helped Mark explore the anxiety and sense of responsibility that drove his need to improve Jennifer's methods. Mark discovered that his perfectionism wasn't really about being right—it was about managing his fear that poor outcomes would reflect badly on him or harm his family.

Jennifer explored her feelings of inadequacy and loss of autonomy. She realized that her withdrawal wasn't just about Mark's criticism— it was about protecting her sense of competence when she felt constantly evaluated.

Phase 3: New interaction patterns (Sessions 13-18)

With better understanding of their underlying emotions, Mark and Jennifer practiced new ways of interacting:

Mark learned to: Recognize his anxiety about suboptimal outcomes, share his concerns without insisting on implementation, ask permission before offering suggestions, and appreciate Jennifer's competence even when her methods differed from his preferences.

Jennifer learned to: Recognize when she was taking Mark's suggestions personally, appreciate his expertise while maintaining her autonomy, communicate her needs for independence clearly, and ask for Mark's input when she genuinely wanted his perspective.

Phase 4: Integration and maintenance (Sessions 19-24)

The final phase focused on practicing their new patterns consistently and developing strategies for handling setbacks. Mark and Jennifer created agreements about when Mark's optimization was welcome and when Jennifer needed space for her own approaches.

Breakthrough moments:

Session 8: Mark realized that his constant improvements weren't actually making Jennifer happier or their household more harmonious. "I thought I was helping her be more successful, but I was actually making her feel less confident."

Session 14: Jennifer recognized that she could appreciate Mark's expertise without feeling obligated to adopt all his suggestions. "I can say, 'That's a great idea, and I'm going to stick with my approach' without it being a rejection of him."

Session 20: Both partners experienced their first conflict resolution that ended with both people feeling heard and satisfied with the outcome. They disagreed about vacation planning approaches and found a compromise that utilized Mark's research skills and Jennifer's spontaneity preferences.

Current relationship dynamic:

Three years post-therapy, Mark and Jennifer describe their marriage as stronger than it's ever been. They still have different approaches to tasks and decisions, but they've learned to appreciate these differences as complementary rather than problematic.

Mark's perspective: "I still notice ways things could be done more efficiently, but I don't feel compelled to fix everything. Jennifer has excellent judgment, and her approaches often work better for her personality and priorities than my methods would."

Jennifer's perspective: "I know Mark's suggestions come from caring rather than criticism. I can choose which input to use and which to set aside without feeling like I'm disappointing him or proving I'm incompetent."

Their practical agreements:

- Mark handles financial planning, travel research, and major purchase decisions where his thoroughness provides clear benefits

- Jennifer manages social planning, home decorating, and creative projects where her flexibility and intuition work better

- Both consult each other about decisions but respect the primary decision-maker's final choice

- They have code words for when optimization pressure is getting overwhelming or when input would be appreciated

Keys to their therapy success:

Both partners were motivated to improve their relationship and willing to examine their own contributions to negative patterns.

The therapist understood OCPD and could help Mark develop insight without pathologizing his conscientiousness.

Focus on interaction patterns rather than individual personality changes made the work feel manageable and relevant.

Practical skill development gave them concrete tools for handling perfectionist pressure and communication challenges.

Sufficient session commitment allowed time for deep pattern change rather than surface-level adjustments.

Ongoing practice of new skills outside sessions helped integrate changes into daily life.

The boundary victory: Partner who reclaimed their identity

When Maria first started dating Carlos, she admired his attention to detail, his organizational skills, and his dedication to excellence. Five years into their marriage, those same qualities had created a dynamic where Maria felt like she was losing herself in Carlos's optimization of every aspect of their shared life.

"I couldn't make a simple decision without wondering what Carlos would think was the better choice," Maria explains. "I'd started shopping for groceries with his preferences in mind, decorating our home according to his aesthetic standards, and even choosing my clothes based on what he considered most flattering. I realized I had no idea what I actually liked anymore."

The turning point came when Maria attended a support group for partners of people with personality disorders and heard other people describe similar experiences of identity erosion. She realized that loving someone with perfectionist tendencies didn't require abandoning her own preferences and approaches.

Maria's boundary journey:

Phase 1: Recognizing the problem (Months 1-2)

Maria started paying attention to how many decisions she was making based on Carlos's standards rather than her own preferences. She was shocked to discover that she rarely chose restaurants, movies, vacation destinations, or even weekend activities without first considering what Carlos would consider optimal.

She began keeping a journal of moments when she automatically deferred to Carlos's judgment and moments when she wanted to assert her own preferences but chose not to avoid conflict or lengthy discussions about better alternatives.

Phase 2: Rediscovering personal preferences (Months 3-4)

Maria started experimenting with making choices based purely on what she wanted rather than what would produce the best outcomes. She bought coffee from a convenient but not optimal shop. She chose outfits she liked rather than ones Carlos considered most flattering. She planned a weekend activity that sounded fun to her without researching whether better options were available.

These small experiments helped Maria reconnect with her own decision-making process and reminded her that she had good judgment and valid preferences.

Phase 3: Implementing boundaries (Months 5-8)

Maria began using the boundary techniques described in Chapter 4, stating clearly what she would do while acknowledging Carlos's right to his different preferences:

"I'm going to choose the restaurant for tonight, and you're welcome to suggest alternatives if you'd like to pick next time."

"I appreciate that you've found a more efficient route, and I prefer this way for the scenery."

"I can see you have ideas about better organization systems, and I'm satisfied with my current approach."

Initially, Carlos was confused and somewhat hurt by Maria's new assertiveness. He genuinely believed his suggestions were helpful and couldn't understand why she was suddenly resistant to obviously beneficial improvements.

Phase 4: Relationship renegotiation (Months 9-12)

As Maria maintained her boundaries consistently, she and Carlos began developing new patterns of interaction. Carlos learned to ask whether Maria wanted suggestions rather than automatically providing them. Maria learned to appreciate Carlos's expertise while maintaining her decision-making autonomy.

They created agreements about areas where Carlos's optimization was welcome (financial planning, home maintenance, major purchases) and areas where Maria wanted independence (daily decisions, personal choices, creative projects).

Current relationship dynamic:

Two years after beginning her boundary work, Maria describes feeling like herself again while still benefiting from her partnership with Carlos.

Maria's transformation:

Confidence restored: "I trust my own judgment again. I can make decisions quickly without second-guessing myself or needing Carlos's approval."

Identity clarity: "I know what I like, what matters to me, and what my priorities are. I'm not trying to optimize everything—I'm living according to my values."

Relationship appreciation: "I love Carlos's thoroughness and expertise, but now I appreciate it as his strength rather than feeling like I have to adopt his approach to everything."

Reduced resentment: "I'm not angry about his suggestions anymore because I don't feel pressured to follow them. I can hear his input and choose what's useful to me."

Carlos's adjustments:

Increased respect: "I've learned that Maria has excellent judgment even when her methods are different from mine. Her approaches often work better for her personality and priorities."

Reduced anxiety: "I don't feel responsible for optimizing Maria's decisions anymore. I can offer input when she wants it, but I don't have to worry about suboptimal outcomes in areas she's handling."

Better appreciation: "I see Maria's strengths more clearly now—her creativity, her ability to make quick decisions, her social intuition. These aren't areas where my optimization helps."

Their practical systems:

Decision ownership: Each person has primary authority over certain life areas, with input from the other welcome but not required.

Suggestion protocols: Carlos asks "Would you like suggestions about this?" before offering optimization ideas.

Appreciation practices: They regularly acknowledge each other's different strengths rather than focusing on areas for improvement.

Time boundaries: Discussions about methods or approaches have agreed-upon time limits to prevent optimization from taking over their conversations.

Individual space: Both partners maintain activities, friendships, and interests that reflect their personal preferences rather than joint optimization.

Keys to Maria's boundary success:

Individual therapy helped Maria develop insight into how she'd lost touch with her own preferences and gave her strategies for reclaiming her identity.

Support group participation provided validation that her experiences were common in perfectionist relationships and that change was possible.

Gradual implementation of boundaries allowed both partners to adjust to new patterns without creating crisis or ultimatums.

Consistency in maintaining boundaries even when Carlos was confused or resistant to the changes.

Both/And thinking that allowed Maria to appreciate Carlos's strengths while maintaining her own approaches.

Self-compassion for the time it took to rediscover her preferences and rebuild her confidence in her own judgment.

Focus on personal growth rather than trying to change Carlos's perfectionist tendencies.

Maria's story illustrates that it's possible to reclaim your identity and autonomy even in relationships with strong perfectionist dynamics. The key is recognizing that loving someone doesn't require abandoning your own judgment and preferences.

The conscious uncoupling: Peaceful separation stories

Not all OCPD relationships end in reconciliation and improved dynamics. Sometimes the kindest and healthiest choice for everyone involved is separation that preserves mutual respect while allowing both partners to find situations that better match their needs.

David and Susan's story:

After eight years of marriage and two children, David and Susan reached a mutual understanding that their fundamental approaches to life were creating more stress than joy for both of them, despite their genuine love and respect for each other.

David thrived on structure, planning, and optimization. He felt most comfortable when systems were in place, decisions were thoroughly researched, and outcomes were carefully controlled. Susan was naturally spontaneous, creative, and flexible. She felt most alive when she could follow her intuition, embrace unexpected opportunities, and accept imperfect outcomes.

For years, they'd tried to bridge their differences. David had worked on becoming more flexible, and Susan had tried to appreciate structure and planning. But their core needs remained incompatible in ways that created ongoing tension.

"We realized that we were both good people trying to fit into lifestyles that didn't suit us," Susan explains. "David needed a partner who appreciated systematic approaches, and I needed someone who enjoyed spontaneous adventures."

Their separation process:

Mutual decision: Rather than one partner leaving the other, David and Susan made the decision together after extensive couples therapy helped them understand that their differences weren't problems to be solved but fundamental incompatibilities.

Professional guidance: They worked with a mediator and therapist throughout the separation process to ensure they were making decisions that protected everyone's wellbeing, especially their children's.

Gradual transition: Instead of abrupt separation, they spent six months transitioning to independent living while maintaining family stability and positive interaction.

Children-focused planning: Their primary concern was helping their children understand and adjust to the changes while maintaining strong relationships with both parents.

Respectful communication: They committed to speaking positively about each other to their children and to others, focusing on compatibility issues rather than blaming or criticizing.

Current co-parenting relationship:

Three years after their divorce, David and Susan have created a co-parenting partnership that works well for everyone involved.

David's perspective: "Susan is an excellent mother, and our children benefit enormously from her creativity and spontaneity. I can appreciate those qualities in her parenting even though they didn't work well in our marriage."

Susan's perspective: "David provides our kids with structure and stability that complements what I offer. They're lucky to have both perspectives in their lives."

Their children's adjustment:

Both children, now 12 and 15, have adapted well to their parents' divorce and report feeling loved and supported by both parents.

Older son: "It's actually less stressful now because Mom and Dad aren't trying to change each other anymore. Dad helps me with organization and planning, and Mom helps me with creative projects and social stuff."

Younger daughter: "I like having two homes because they're different. Dad's house is really organized and peaceful, and Mom's house is more relaxed and fun. I need both."

Practical arrangements:

Shared custody: The children spend equal time with both parents but can request adjustments based on their needs and preferences.

Complementary strengths: David handles structured activities, academic support, and financial planning. Susan manages creative activities, social events, and emotional support.

Consistent communication: David and Susan meet monthly to coordinate parenting decisions and maintain consistency in rules and expectations.

Mutual support: They attend school events together, celebrate children's achievements jointly, and consult each other about parenting challenges.

Individual growth: Both parents have found new partners who better match their lifestyles and approaches to life.

Tom and Rachel's story:

Tom and Rachel's marriage ended after Rachel developed severe depression and anxiety related to living with Tom's perfectionist demands. Despite therapy and medication, Rachel's mental health continued to deteriorate under the pressure of constant optimization and criticism.

"I loved Tom, but I was disappearing," Rachel explains. "I couldn't handle the daily pressure of having every decision analyzed and every method improved. I needed space to heal."

Tom initially resisted the separation, believing they could solve their problems through better communication and system optimization. But Rachel's deteriorating mental health made it clear that the relationship dynamic was genuinely harmful to her wellbeing.

Their healing process:

Individual therapy: Both partners worked extensively with therapists to process their relationship experiences and develop healthier approaches to future relationships.

Rachel's recovery: With space from perfectionist pressure, Rachel's mental health improved significantly. She rediscovered her confidence, rebuilt her social connections, and developed career goals.

Tom's insight: Through therapy, Tom began understanding how his OCPD created genuine distress for others, even when his intentions were helpful. He developed strategies for managing his perfectionist tendencies.

Respectful distance: They maintained cordial but limited contact, focusing on practical matters and avoiding rehashing relationship issues.

Current status:

Five years post-divorce, both Tom and Rachel have rebuilt their lives successfully.

Rachel's perspective: "Leaving was the hardest decision I've ever made, but it saved my mental health and probably my life. I'm grateful for the good years we had, and I'm glad we both found peace."

Tom's perspective: "I didn't understand how my behavior affected Rachel until after she left. I wish I'd developed that insight earlier, but I've learned from the experience and I'm working to be a better partner in future relationships."

Keys to peaceful separation:

Mutual respect for each other's needs and wellbeing rather than blame or criticism.

Professional support to navigate the emotional and practical challenges of separation.

Focus on learning rather than trying to determine who was right or wrong.

Commitment to individual growth and development rather than remaining stuck in relationship dynamics.

Children-first approach when kids are involved, prioritizing their wellbeing over parental preferences.

Realistic expectations about what separation can and cannot accomplish.

These stories illustrate that conscious uncoupling can be a loving choice when fundamental incompatibilities create unsustainable stress for one or both partners. Sometimes the kindest thing couples can do is acknowledge that they're not right for each other while preserving respect and appreciation for what they did share.

Common elements in successful outcomes

Whether OCPD relationships improve through medication, therapy, boundaries, or conscious separation, certain factors appear consistently in positive outcomes.

Both partners take responsibility for their contributions to relationship dynamics rather than blaming each other for problems.

Professional support provides objective guidance and evidence-based strategies that couples can't develop on their own.

Realistic expectations about change focus on improving dynamics rather than expecting personality transformation.

Individual growth happens alongside relationship work, with both partners developing better self-awareness and coping skills.

Long-term commitment to improvement recognizes that meaningful change takes time and consistent effort.

Focus on strengths alongside problem-solving helps partners remember why they care about each other and their relationship.

Flexibility about outcomes allows couples to discover solutions that work for their specific situation rather than following predetermined models.

Children's wellbeing remains the priority when kids are involved, influencing decisions about staying together or separating.

Respect for differences develops over time, with partners learning to appreciate rather than trying to eliminate their different approaches.

Support systems provide perspective, encouragement, and practical assistance throughout the change process.

Hope balanced with realism

These success stories provide genuine hope for OCPD relationships, but they also illustrate the significant effort required for positive outcomes. Change is possible, but it's not easy, quick, or guaranteed.

What these stories demonstrate:

OCPD symptoms can be managed effectively with appropriate treatment, allowing for more flexible and collaborative relationships.

Partners can learn to appreciate each other's different strengths rather than trying to optimize each other into similarity.

Children can benefit from exposure to both structured and flexible approaches to life when parents work together effectively.

Sometimes the most loving choice is separation that allows both partners to find more compatible situations.

Individual growth and professional support are usually necessary components of relationship improvement.

Small, consistent changes often produce better results than dramatic attempts at transformation.

What these stories don't promise:

Easy solutions or quick fixes for deeply ingrained personality patterns.

Complete elimination of perfectionist tendencies or standards.

Relationships that never experience conflict or tension.

Universal approaches that work for every OCPD partnership.

Change without significant investment of time, effort, and often financial resources.

Success without both partners being motivated to work on improvement.

Realistic hope for your situation:

If you're living with OCPD relationship challenges, these stories suggest several possibilities for positive outcomes:

Your partner may benefit from medication that reduces the anxiety driving their need for control.

Therapy can help both of you develop better communication and conflict resolution skills.

Boundaries can protect your mental health while allowing you to appreciate your partner's strengths.

Your relationship may improve significantly with consistent effort and professional support.

If your relationship can't be saved, you may still be able to separate peacefully and maintain respect for each other.

Your children can thrive regardless of whether you stay together or separate, as long as their needs remain the priority.

You can reclaim your identity and confidence even if you've lost touch with yourself in the relationship.

The key is matching your expectations to your specific situation, being realistic about what's required for change, and committing to whatever path you choose with full investment rather than half-hearted effort.

Creating your own success story

Whatever direction your relationship takes, you have the power to create positive outcomes by focusing on what you can control and getting appropriate support for the challenges you face.

If you're working on improving your relationship:

Invest in professional help rather than trying to solve complex personality disorder issues on your own.

Focus on your own growth and responses rather than trying to change your partner's fundamental personality.

Celebrate small improvements rather than waiting for dramatic transformation.

Maintain your individual identity and support systems throughout the improvement process.

Set realistic timelines for seeing changes and be prepared for setbacks along the way.

If you're considering separation:

Get professional guidance to help you make informed decisions and navigate the process skillfully.

Focus on your wellbeing and your children's needs rather than trying to punish or change your partner.

Build your support systems and develop independence gradually rather than making impulsive decisions.

Consider all options including trial separation, individual therapy, and mediated separation before making final choices.

Prepare financially and emotionally for the transition rather than leaving in crisis mode.

Regardless of your path:

Take care of your mental health through therapy, self-care, and support systems.

Trust your judgment about what you can and cannot accept in relationships.

Focus on what you've learned rather than viewing relationship challenges as failures.

Maintain hope for positive outcomes while being realistic about what change requires.

Remember that you deserve to feel valued, respected, and emotionally safe in your relationships.

Your story doesn't have to look exactly like any of the examples in this chapter. The path forward depends on your specific circumstances, your partner's willingness to grow, and your own values and priorities. But these stories demonstrate that positive change is possible, whether that means healing your relationship or healing yourself through separation.

Real hope through diverse pathways to resolution

The success stories in this chapter illustrate that there isn't one right way to address OCPD relationship challenges. Medication helped David manage his anxiety about imperfection. Therapy gave Mark and Jennifer new tools for connection and communication. Boundaries allowed Maria to reclaim her identity while staying in her marriage. Conscious separation enabled David, Susan, Tom, and Rachel to find peace and respect despite incompatibility.

What all these stories share is commitment to growth, realistic expectations about change, professional support, and respect for everyone's wellbeing. They demonstrate that OCPD relationships can have positive outcomes, but those outcomes require insight, effort, and often significant support to achieve.

Most importantly, these stories show that you don't have to accept a relationship that diminishes your mental health or sense of self. Whether through improving your current relationship or finding the courage to leave an unsustainable situation, you have options for creating a life that honors your needs and values.

Your story of resolution and growth is still being written. With the right support, realistic expectations, and commitment to your own wellbeing, you can create outcomes that seemed impossible when you first picked up this book.

Chapter 11: Rediscovering who you were before the criticism

Lisa found the box buried in her closet behind winter coats she hadn't worn in years. Inside, she discovered pieces of herself she'd forgotten existed: sketches from an art class she'd taken five years ago, business cards from networking events she'd attended with enthusiasm, photos from hiking trips with friends she rarely saw anymore, and a journal filled with dreams and goals that felt like they belonged to a different person.

As she sat on her bedroom floor surrounded by these artifacts of her former self, Lisa realized she couldn't pinpoint exactly when she'd stopped drawing, stopped networking, stopped hiking, or stopped dreaming. The changes had been gradual—each interest quietly abandoned as her husband Mark's standards and opinions slowly reshaped how she spent her time and energy.

"I used to be interesting," she whispered to herself, holding a sketch that demonstrated real talent. "I used to have opinions about things. I used to make decisions without wondering what Mark would think."

The woman who had created these sketches felt confident about her artistic ability. The person who had attended those networking events believed her career ideas had merit. The hiker in those photos trusted her judgment about trails, weather, and adventure. But somewhere along the way, living with Mark's perfectionism had convinced Lisa that her instincts were unreliable, her interests weren't productive enough, and her dreams needed optimization to be worth pursuing.

Lisa's discovery represents a turning point many OCPD partners experience—the moment they realize they've lost touch with fundamental aspects of themselves while adapting to someone else's standards and expectations. The person they were before the relationship feels like a stranger, buried under years of second-guessing, self-editing, and gradual erosion of personal autonomy.

But here's the encouraging truth: **that person isn't gone.** They're simply covered up by layers of adaptation and self-doubt. Rediscovering who you were before the criticism isn't about rejecting your current life or relationship—it's about reclaiming the parts of yourself that make you feel alive, confident, and genuinely you.

Identity reconstruction after years of control

Living with someone whose standards dominate household decisions creates a subtle but profound form of identity erosion. You don't lose yourself all at once—it happens through thousands of small moments where your natural inclinations are redirected toward more optimal approaches.

Over time, this process can leave you feeling disconnected from your authentic preferences, unsure of your judgment, and unclear about what actually brings you joy versus what you've learned to appreciate because it meets external standards.

Understanding identity erosion patterns:

Preference confusion occurs when you've adapted to someone else's standards for so long that you can't distinguish between what you genuinely like and what you've learned to accept as "better" choices. You might find yourself ordering food your partner would approve of, choosing clothes they consider flattering, or planning activities they would find worthwhile without conscious awareness that you're filtering your preferences through their lens.

Decision paralysis develops when you've received so much input about "better" ways to approach choices that you can't make simple decisions without anxiety about whether you're doing it right. The grocery store becomes overwhelming when you're evaluating every purchase against optimization criteria that aren't even your own.

Interest abandonment happens gradually as hobbies, friendships, and activities that don't align with your partner's values or that they don't understand get deprioritized. You don't consciously decide to stop drawing or hiking or seeing certain friends—you just find that these activities create friction or lengthy discussions about better uses of time.

Goal suppression occurs when your dreams and ambitions get filtered through someone else's analysis of what's realistic, practical, or likely to succeed. You may stop mentioning ideas that seem to trigger your partner's problem-solving mode or that they evaluate as inefficient uses of resources.

Personality flattening results from years of self-editing to avoid triggering perfectionist anxiety in your partner. Your humor becomes more careful, your spontaneity decreases, and your natural emotional expressiveness gets muted to maintain household harmony.

Research shows that partners of individuals with controlling personality traits often experience significant identity confusion and loss of personal agency (Lafreniere & Byers, 2012). This isn't weakness or codependency—it's a natural response to living in an environment where your authentic self creates tension while adaptation brings peace.

The identity reconstruction process involves three stages:

Recognition that you've lost touch with aspects of yourself and acknowledgment that this loss isn't your fault or a sign of personal weakness.

Exploration of who you were before your identity became filtered through someone else's standards, and experimentation with rediscovering those qualities.

Integration of your authentic self with your current life in ways that honor both your individual needs and your relationship commitments.

This process isn't about rejecting everything you've learned or adapted during your relationship. Some changes may reflect genuine growth and positive influence from your partner. But healthy adaptation enhances who you are rather than replacing who you are.

Reconnecting with abandoned interests and friendships

One of the most telling signs of identity erosion in OCPD relationships is the gradual disappearance of activities, relationships, and interests that once brought you energy and joy. These losses often happen so incrementally that you don't notice until you're asked about hobbies and realize you can't think of any, or invited to social events and realize you've lost touch with most of your friends.

Mapping what you've lost:

Interest archaeology involves systematically examining what you used to enjoy before your relationship began or during the early stages when your partner's standards hadn't yet reshaped your choices.

Look through old photos, journal entries, social media posts from several years ago, or conversations with longtime friends about activities you used to share. Create a list of interests, hobbies, and activities that once engaged you, regardless of whether they seem practical or optimal now.

Friendship audit requires honest assessment of social connections that have weakened or disappeared. Identify people you used to enjoy spending time with, colleagues you connected with, or acquaintances who shared your interests. Notice patterns in which relationships have faded and which ones you've maintained.

Dream inventory involves reconnecting with goals, aspirations, and possibilities you used to consider before they were analyzed for practicality or efficiency. What did you want to be, do, or experience before those dreams went through someone else's optimization filter?

Energy tracking helps you identify what activities or experiences used to make you feel alive, creative, or fulfilled. These aren't necessarily things you were good at or that produced measurable outcomes—they're simply activities that energized you.

Common patterns of abandonment:

Creative activities often disappear first because they don't produce measurable outcomes and can seem inefficient compared to more practical uses of time. Drawing, music, writing, crafting, dancing, or other artistic pursuits may have been gradually replaced with activities that your partner considers more worthwhile.

Social connections tend to fade when friends don't meet your partner's standards for interesting conversation, productive activities, or efficient use of social time. You may have stopped seeing people whose approaches to life create tension or whose priorities your partner doesn't understand.

Physical activities might have been abandoned if they seemed inefficient, unsafe, or less optimal than your partner's preferred forms of exercise. Hiking, dancing, pickup sports, or fitness classes may have been replaced with more systematic or measurable approaches to staying healthy.

Professional development in areas that don't align with your partner's career optimization might have been deprioritized. You may have stopped pursuing networking opportunities, creative projects, or skill development that didn't fit your partner's analysis of your most promising career path.

Spontaneous experiences likely decreased as your household became more planned and systematic. Road trips, last-minute events, or unscheduled activities may feel too chaotic or inefficient to suggest anymore.

Strategies for reconnection:

Start small and private to avoid triggering your partner's optimization instincts while you're rediscovering what you actually enjoy. Try activities when your partner isn't around, or engage in interests that don't require explanation or justification.

Give yourself permission to be bad at things you used to enjoy. Years away from creative activities, sports, or hobbies means your skills may be rusty, and that's completely normal. Focus on enjoyment rather than performance.

Reach out gradually to friends you've lost touch with. Start with low-pressure contact—social media messages, brief texts, or casual invitations—rather than trying to immediately resume intensive friendships.

Experiment with new versions of old interests. If you used to paint, try digital art or art classes. If you enjoyed hiking, start with nature walks or indoor rock climbing. Allow your interests to adapt to your current life while preserving their essential appeal.

Create separate space for these activities so they don't become subject to household optimization. This might mean joining groups that meet outside your home, pursuing interests during times when your partner is occupied elsewhere, or simply establishing that certain activities are yours to manage independently.

Overcoming learned helplessness and decision paralysis

Years of having your choices improved, corrected, or taken over can create a pattern where you doubt your ability to make good decisions independently. This learned helplessness isn't about lack of intelligence or capability—it's about adaptation to an environment where your natural decision-making process has been consistently redirected.

Understanding decision paralysis patterns:

Analysis overwhelm occurs when you've absorbed your partner's thorough approach to decision-making and now feel anxious making choices without extensive research and comparison. Simple decisions like choosing a restaurant or buying household items become complex projects requiring optimization.

Perfectionism anxiety develops when you've internalized impossibly high standards for outcomes and fear making choices that won't meet these criteria. You may procrastinate on decisions rather than risk choosing suboptimal options.

Approval seeking becomes automatic when you've gotten used to running decisions by your partner for input or validation. You may find yourself mentally asking "What would they think?" even for choices that don't affect them.

Confidence erosion happens gradually as repeated corrections and improvements convince you that your instincts aren't reliable. You may second-guess choices you feel good about or assume others know better approaches.

Responsibility avoidance can develop as a protective strategy when making decisions leads to analysis, criticism, or takeover. You may defer choices to others rather than risking the stress of having your approach evaluated.

Rebuilding decision-making confidence:

Start with low-stakes choices where the consequences of suboptimal decisions are minimal. Choose your lunch, your route to work, your weekend activities, or your entertainment without consulting anyone else or doing extensive research.

Practice "good enough" decision-making by consciously choosing options that meet your needs without being optimal. This helps retrain your brain to accept adequate outcomes rather than requiring perfect choices.

Set decision timelines to prevent endless analysis. Give yourself specific time limits for choosing restaurants, making purchases, or selecting activities. Honor these timelines even if you haven't found the theoretically best option.

Track successful decisions by keeping a journal of choices that worked out well, even if they weren't optimal. This creates evidence that your judgment is more reliable than your self-doubt suggests.

Notice your preferences before analyzing them. When faced with choices, pay attention to your initial instinct or emotional response before your analytical mind takes over. This gut reaction often contains valuable information about what you actually want.

Celebrate imperfect outcomes that still meet your needs. When your restaurant choice is decent but not amazing, or your purchase works fine but isn't the best possible option, practice feeling satisfied with adequate rather than disappointed about missed optimization.

Gradual independence building:

Week 1-2: Make three small decisions daily without consultation or research. Choose what to wear, what to have for breakfast, which route to take somewhere.

Week 3-4: Extend to slightly bigger decisions like where to shop, what movie to watch, or how to spend a free afternoon. Practice accepting outcomes without comparing them to potentially better alternatives.

Week 5-6: Take on decisions that affect household functioning but don't require your partner's input, like organizing your personal spaces, choosing gifts for your family, or planning individual activities.

Week 7-8: Make financial decisions within agreed-upon parameters, such as choosing restaurants, making personal purchases, or selecting services like haircuts or car maintenance.

Week 9-10: Plan activities that involve other people, like social events, family outings, or shared meals, while accepting input but maintaining decision-making authority.

Week 11-12: Take on bigger decisions that affect your personal goals and development, such as career moves, educational opportunities, or major life changes.

The confidence rebuilding program (12-week guide)

Systematic confidence rebuilding requires consistent practice and gradual challenge escalation. This 12-week program helps you redevelop trust in your judgment while building evidence of your capability and worth.

Week 1-2: Foundation Building

Daily practices:

- Make three decisions without consulting anyone (clothing, food, routes)

- Notice one thing you handle competently each day

- Spend 15 minutes on an activity you choose purely for enjoyment

- Practice saying "I prefer" instead of "I don't know" when asked about preferences

Week 2 goals:

- Reduce automatic approval-seeking for minor decisions

- Begin recognizing your natural preferences and instincts

- Build evidence that your choices can produce acceptable outcomes

- Start distinguishing between your voice and internalized criticism

Week 3-4: Preference Exploration

Daily practices:

- Try one new thing based purely on curiosity or interest
- Express an opinion without immediately qualifying or softening it
- Choose entertainment, food, or activities based on what appeals to you
- Notice when you're filtering preferences through others' standards

Week 4 goals:

- Develop clearer sense of your authentic likes and dislikes
- Reduce hesitation about expressing preferences
- Build comfort with choosing based on personal appeal rather than optimal outcomes
- Strengthen connection to your intuitive responses

Week 5-6: Social Confidence

Daily practices:

- Initiate one social interaction (text, call, invitation) based on your interest
- Share an opinion in conversation without extensive justification
- Make social plans that reflect your preferences for timing, location, or activity
- Practice saying no to invitations that don't appeal to you

Week 6 goals:

- Rebuild social initiative and relationship ownership

- Develop comfort with being seen as you authentically are
- Strengthen ability to maintain your position in social discussions
- Reduce people-pleasing in favor of genuine connection

Week 7-8: Creative and Personal Expression

Daily practices:

- Engage in creative activity without concern for skill level or outcome
- Express yourself through clothing, decoration, or personal style choices
- Share something you've created, learned, or experienced with others
- Practice receiving feedback without immediately agreeing or defending

Week 8 goals:

- Reconnect with creative and expressive aspects of your personality
- Build tolerance for imperfection in your creative efforts
- Develop comfort with being visible in your authentic interests and style
- Strengthen resilience to criticism or feedback

Week 9-10: Professional and Goal-Oriented Confidence

Daily practices:

- Take initiative on one work or personal project without extensive planning

- Apply for opportunities, make connections, or pursue goals based on interest rather than guaranteed success

- Share your professional or personal goals with others without apologizing for ambition

- Practice advocating for yourself in professional or goal-oriented contexts

Week 10 goals:

- Rebuild professional and personal ambition

- Develop comfort with taking calculated risks

- Strengthen ability to promote yourself and your capabilities

- Reduce perfectionist paralysis in goal pursuit

Week 11-12: Integration and Future Planning

Daily practices:

- Make decisions that integrate your rediscovered preferences with your current life responsibilities

- Set goals and make plans that reflect your authentic interests and values

- Communicate your needs and boundaries clearly in important relationships

- Practice maintaining your sense of self during challenging or stressful situations

Week 12 goals:

- Integrate authentic self with current life circumstances

- Develop sustainable practices for maintaining confidence and identity

- Create clear vision for your future that reflects your values and desires
- Build resilience for ongoing identity maintenance in challenging relationships

Confidence indicators to track:

Decision-making speed: How quickly can you make routine decisions without anxiety or extensive analysis?

Preference clarity: How easily can you identify what you want, like, or prefer in various situations?

Opinion expression: How comfortable are you sharing your thoughts and perspectives without extensive qualification?

Goal pursuit: How willing are you to pursue interests and ambitions despite potential criticism or imperfection?

Social initiative: How often do you initiate social contact, make plans, or suggest activities based on your preferences?

Boundary maintenance: How consistently can you maintain your limits and needs despite pressure or guilt?

Creative risk-taking: How willing are you to try new things, make mistakes, or show others your imperfect efforts?

Self-advocacy: How effectively can you promote your needs, interests, and capabilities in various contexts?

Identity Reclamation Workbook

This workbook provides structured exercises for systematically rediscovering and reclaiming aspects of yourself that may have been lost or suppressed during your relationship.

Part 1: Identity Archaeology

Exercise 1: The Person I Used to Be

Write detailed descriptions of yourself during different life periods:

- High school/college: What did you enjoy? What were your goals? How did you spend free time?

- Early adulthood: What excited you? What did you think you'd become? What brought you energy?

- Before your current relationship: What were your interests, friendships, and ambitions like?

- Early in your relationship: What aspects of yourself did your partner initially find attractive?

Exercise 2: Interest Inventory

Create comprehensive lists in each category:

Creative interests I used to have: (art, music, writing, crafting, etc.) **Physical activities I enjoyed:** (sports, hiking, dancing, fitness classes, etc.) **Social activities that energized me:** (parties, clubs, networking, community involvement, etc.) **Learning interests I pursued:** (languages, skills, subjects, certifications, etc.) **Career goals I used to have:** (positions, industries, projects, entrepreneurial ideas, etc.)

Exercise 3: Friendship Mapping

Identify relationships that have changed:

- Friends I've lost touch with and miss

- Colleagues I used to connect with more

- Family members I see less often

- Social groups or communities I've drifted away from

- People who knew me before I changed

Part 2: Values and Preferences Clarification

Exercise 4: Value Identification

Rank these values in order of personal importance to you:

- Achievement/Success
- Adventure/Excitement
- Authenticity/Being genuine
- Beauty/Aesthetics
- Community/Belonging
- Creativity/Self-expression
- Family/Relationships
- Freedom/Independence
- Fun/Enjoyment
- Growth/Learning
- Health/Wellness
- Justice/Fairness
- Knowledge/Understanding
- Leadership/Influence
- Peace/Harmony
- Security/Stability
- Service/Helping others
- Spirituality/Meaning

Exercise 5: Preference Exploration

Complete these statements with your first instinct, before analyzing:

- I feel most energized when I'm...
- I feel most like myself when I'm...

- I'm happiest when I'm surrounded by...

- I feel most confident when I'm...

- I feel most creative when I'm...

- I'm most relaxed when I'm...

- I feel most connected when I'm...

- I'm most excited when I'm...

Exercise 6: Dream Reconstruction

Write about goals and dreams without editing for practicality:

- If money weren't an issue, I would...

- If I weren't afraid of failing, I would try...

- If I could be anything, I would be...

- If I had unlimited time, I would learn...

- If I could live anywhere, I would choose...

- If I could change one thing about my life, it would be...

Part 3: Reconnection Planning

Exercise 7: Interest Revival Strategy

For each abandoned interest you want to explore:

Interest: _____ **Why it used to matter to me:**
_____ **Why I stopped:** _____ **How I could
try it again:** _____ **First small step:**
_____ **Potential obstacles:** _____ **Support
I need:** _____

Exercise 8: Friendship Reconnection Plan

For each relationship you want to rebuild:

Person: _____ What I valued about this relationship: _____ Why we lost touch: _____ First contact approach: _____ Realistic expectation for renewed connection: _____ How this relationship supports my authentic self: _____

Exercise 9: Identity Integration Goals

Areas where I want to be more authentic: _____ Changes I want to make in how I express myself: _____ Boundaries I need to maintain my sense of self: _____ Support systems I need to build: _____ Timeline for identity integration: _____

Part 4: Progress Tracking

Exercise 10: Weekly Identity Check-ins

Each week, assess:

- Moments when I felt most like myself

- Decisions I made based on my authentic preferences

- Times I expressed my genuine opinions or feelings

- Activities that brought me energy and joy

- Relationships that supported my authentic self

- Progress toward my identity integration goals

Exercise 11: Monthly Identity Assessment

Rate your progress monthly (1-10 scale):

- Clarity about my preferences and values

- Comfort expressing my authentic self

- Confidence in my decision-making

- Connection to my interests and passions

- Quality of my supportive relationships

- Overall sense of being true to myself

Exercise 12: Identity Maintenance Planning

Develop sustainable practices for maintaining your authentic self:

- Daily practices that keep me connected to who I am

- Weekly activities that energize and fulfill me

- Monthly check-ins with supportive friends or professionals

- Quarterly reviews of my goals and values

- Annual assessment of my identity integration progress

Working with resistance from your partner

As you rediscover and express your authentic self, you may encounter resistance, confusion, or concern from your OCPD partner. They've become accustomed to the adapted version of you and may experience your changes as threatening or problematic.

Common partner reactions:

Confusion about your changes: "You never used to be interested in art classes. Why are you starting now?" **Concern about time management:** "Don't you think that time could be better spent on more practical activities?" **Anxiety about your independence:** "I don't understand why you need to make these decisions without discussing them with me." **Criticism of your choices:** "That friend/activity/interest doesn't seem very beneficial for your goals."

Strategies for managing partner resistance:

Stay connected to your motivation for identity reclamation. Your partner's discomfort with your changes doesn't mean you should abandon your authentic self.

Use clear communication about what you're doing and why: "I'm reconnecting with parts of myself that I've missed. This isn't about rejecting you or our relationship—it's about being a more complete person."

Set appropriate boundaries around your identity exploration: "This is something I'm doing for my own growth. I appreciate your concern, and I'm going to continue with this."

Invite positive engagement when appropriate: "I'd love to share what I'm learning in my art class, but I'm not looking for suggestions about how to do it differently."

Stay patient with the adjustment period while maintaining your commitment to change. Your partner may need time to adapt to your increased independence and self-expression.

Building ongoing support systems

Identity reclamation is easier to maintain when you have relationships and environments that support your authentic self rather than requiring constant adaptation to external standards.

Professional support systems:

Individual therapy provides objective guidance for identity exploration and integration, especially with therapists experienced in helping people recover from controlling relationships.

Support groups for partners of people with personality disorders offer validation and practical strategies from others facing similar challenges.

Career counseling can help you reconnect with professional goals and ambitions that may have been suppressed or redirected.

Life coaching provides accountability and encouragement for pursuing goals and making changes that reflect your authentic values.

Personal support systems:

Authentic friendships with people who appreciate you for who you are rather than expecting you to meet external standards.

Interest-based communities through classes, clubs, or groups that support your natural interests and passions.

Family connections with relatives who remember and value your authentic self.

Mentor relationships with people who can guide your growth in areas that matter to you personally.

Environmental supports:

Physical spaces that reflect your aesthetic preferences and support your interests and activities.

Time boundaries that protect space for your authentic interests and self-expression.

Financial independence that allows you to pursue your interests and goals without requiring approval or justification.

Social environments that encourage authenticity, creativity, and individual expression.

The goal isn't to reject your entire current life or relationship, but to ensure that your authentic self has space to exist and grow alongside your other commitments and responsibilities.

Sustaining your authentic identity long-term

Identity reclamation isn't a one-time project—it requires ongoing attention and protection, especially when living with someone whose personality tends toward optimization and control.

Daily identity maintenance practices:

Morning intention setting: Start each day by connecting with your authentic values and goals before adapting to external demands.

Decision ownership: Make several choices daily based on your genuine preferences rather than external optimization.

Creative expression: Engage in activities that allow you to express your authentic self, even in small ways.

Boundary maintenance: Practice protecting your autonomy and identity throughout daily interactions.

Evening reflection: End each day by acknowledging moments when you expressed your authentic self and areas where you want more authenticity tomorrow.

Weekly identity strengthening:

Pursue authentic interests through classes, activities, or hobbies that energize you.

Connect with supportive relationships that appreciate your genuine self.

Practice self-advocacy in situations that matter to your identity and goals.

Assess and adjust your balance between adaptation and authenticity.

Plan activities that reflect your values and bring you genuine satisfaction.

Monthly identity evaluation:

Review your progress toward identity integration goals and adjust your approach as needed.

Assess relationship dynamics to ensure your authentic self is being respected and supported.

Celebrate growth and acknowledge the courage it takes to reclaim your identity.

Plan upcoming activities that will support your continued authenticity and growth.

Seek professional support if you're struggling with identity maintenance or partner resistance.

Your identity reclamation journey is unique to your specific situation, personality, and circumstances. The goal isn't to become someone completely different, but to rediscover and integrate the authentic parts of yourself that have been suppressed or abandoned during your adaptation to someone else's standards.

Systematic approach to recovering your authentic self

The process outlined in this chapter provides a structured pathway for rediscovering who you are beneath the layers of adaptation and optimization. It acknowledges that identity erosion happens gradually and systematically, so identity reclamation also requires systematic, intentional work.

Most importantly, this approach recognizes that you deserve to feel like yourself in your own life. Your preferences, interests, goals, and ways of being in the world have value independent of whether they meet external standards for optimization or efficiency.

Reclaiming your authentic self isn't selfish or disloyal to your relationship. It's necessary for your mental health, your ability to contribute genuinely to your partnerships, and your capacity to model authenticity for any children who are watching you navigate these challenges.

The person you were before the criticism is still there, waiting to be rediscovered and welcomed back into your life. With patience, courage, and systematic effort, you can reconnect with that person while building a life that honors both your authentic self and your current responsibilities and relationships.

Chapter 12: Creating Emotional safety in an unsafe relationship

Amy discovered she had developed what she privately called "hypervigilance mode"—a state of constant alertness about her husband David's mood, stress level, and potential triggers. She could sense from his footsteps on the stairs whether his workday had gone well, predict from his tone during phone calls whether dinner conversation would be pleasant or tense, and gauge from his morning routine whether household interactions would be smooth or filled with corrections.

This hypervigilance wasn't paranoia or oversensitivity. It was an adaptive response to living with someone whose anxiety about imperfection could transform routine family moments into optimization sessions that left everyone feeling tense and inadequate.

Amy found herself mentally cataloguing the state of the house before David came home, anticipating which household management choices might trigger lengthy discussions about better approaches, and emotionally preparing for feedback about decisions she'd made during the day. She was living in a constant state of low-level stress, always ready to manage someone else's emotional responses to imperfection.

But over the past year, Amy had learned something crucial: **she could create internal safety even when external safety felt limited.** Through therapy and her own research, she'd developed strategies for protecting her emotional wellbeing while remaining in a challenging relationship.

Amy's journey toward emotional safety didn't require David to change his perfectionist tendencies or develop sudden flexibility about standards. It required her to develop psychological boundaries, emotional regulation skills, and internal practices that preserved her mental health despite ongoing exposure to criticism and control.

This chapter explores how to build emotional safety from the inside out—creating psychological protection that doesn't depend on your partner's cooperation or insight, while maintaining your ability to function in your relationship and family responsibilities.

Building internal sanctuary when external safety is limited

Emotional safety in relationships typically comes from having a partner who provides empathy, validation, and respect for your feelings and experiences. But OCPD partners often struggle to offer this kind of emotional support because they're focused on solving problems, optimizing outcomes, and managing their own anxiety about imperfection.

When external emotional safety is inconsistent or unavailable, you can develop internal practices that provide stability, validation, and psychological protection regardless of what's happening around you.

Understanding internal sanctuary:

Internal sanctuary isn't about withdrawing from your relationship or family responsibilities. It's about developing psychological resources that remain available to you even when your environment feels critical, chaotic, or emotionally draining.

Think of it as creating a psychological space that exists independently of your partner's moods, reactions, or need for control. This internal space holds your sense of worth, your confidence in your judgment, and your connection to what matters to you personally.

Core components of internal sanctuary:

Self-validation practices help you acknowledge your own experiences and feelings without requiring external confirmation that they're reasonable or justified.

Emotional regulation techniques give you tools for managing your responses to criticism, conflict, or perfectionist pressure without becoming overwhelmed or reactive.

Identity anchoring maintains your connection to who you are beyond your role as your partner's spouse, including your values, interests, and relationships that exist independently of their opinions.

Boundary visualization creates mental separation between your emotional state and your partner's anxiety, frustration, or need to control outcomes.

Meaning-making frameworks help you interpret challenging experiences in ways that support your resilience rather than undermining your sense of competence or worth.

Daily sanctuary practices:

Morning grounding helps you start each day connected to your own emotional center rather than immediately adapting to external demands or moods.

Spend 5-10 minutes before getting out of bed connecting with your breath, setting intentions for your day based on your values, and reminding yourself of your worth and capability. This practice creates an internal foundation that remains accessible throughout the day.

Emotional check-ins throughout the day help you maintain awareness of your feelings and needs rather than becoming completely absorbed in managing others' emotions or reactions.

Set phone reminders to ask yourself: "How am I feeling right now?" "What do I need?" "Am I taking care of myself or just managing others?" These brief pauses help you stay connected to your internal experience.

Validation statements replace the external validation that may be inconsistently available with internal acknowledgment of your experiences.

Practice phrases like: "My feelings make sense given what I'm experiencing," "I'm doing the best I can with a difficult situation," "My reaction is reasonable and understandable," "I deserve respect and kindness."

Evening restoration helps you process the day's experiences and reconnect with your sense of self before sleep.

Spend time acknowledging what you handled well, processing any difficult emotions without trying to fix or change them, and setting intentions for taking care of yourself tomorrow.

Emotional detachment techniques that preserve sanity

Emotional detachment in this context doesn't mean becoming cold or uncaring toward your partner. It means learning to separate your emotional wellbeing from their emotional states, reactions, and need for control.

This kind of healthy detachment preserves your ability to care about your partner while protecting you from becoming overwhelmed by their anxiety, criticism, or perfectionist episodes.

Understanding healthy detachment:

Healthy detachment recognizes that you are not responsible for managing your partner's emotions, reactions, or comfort level with imperfection. You can care about their wellbeing while maintaining boundaries around how much their distress affects your own emotional state.

This is particularly important with OCPD partners because their anxiety about suboptimal outcomes can be intense and compelling. You may feel responsible for reducing their distress by conforming to their standards or avoiding behaviors that trigger their perfectionist anxiety.

But taking responsibility for your partner's emotional comfort often requires sacrificing your own authenticity, autonomy, and emotional wellbeing. Healthy detachment lets you care without caretaking.

Detachment visualization techniques:

The glass wall technique helps you maintain empathy while creating emotional separation. Visualize a clear glass wall between yourself and your partner's emotional intensity. You can see their distress and care about their experience, but their emotions cannot cross the wall to overwhelm your emotional space.

The weather metaphor helps you view your partner's perfectionist episodes as temporary weather patterns that will pass. Their criticism, anxiety, or frustration is like a storm system—intense while it's happening, but not permanent and not a reflection of your worth or capability.

The observer stance involves stepping back mentally to witness your partner's emotional responses rather than being consumed by them. You might think: "I notice that they're feeling frustrated about this inefficiency," rather than "I need to fix this so they feel better."

The separate boats technique visualizes you and your partner as traveling in separate boats on the same river. You're going in the same direction and care about each other's wellbeing, but you're not responsible for steering their boat or preventing them from experiencing rough water.

Practical detachment strategies:

Response delay involves pausing before responding to criticism, corrections, or perfectionist pressure. This pause gives you time to assess your own emotional state and choose a response rather than reacting automatically.

When your partner offers improvements or expresses frustration about suboptimal outcomes, take a breath and ask yourself: "What response serves my wellbeing right now?" rather than automatically trying to reduce their distress.

Emotional labeling helps you recognize and name what you're experiencing without being overwhelmed by it. Practice identifying feelings like: "I notice I'm feeling criticized," "I'm experiencing pressure to conform," "I'm feeling responsible for their comfort."

Energy protection involves consciously choosing how much emotional energy to invest in managing your partner's responses. You might decide: "I'm willing to listen to their concerns, but I'm not willing to spend an hour researching better alternatives," or "I can acknowledge their frustration without taking responsibility for fixing it."

Reframing self-talk replaces automatic thoughts that make you responsible for your partner's emotions with more balanced perspectives:

Instead of: "I need to do this differently so they don't get upset" Try: "They have the right to their feelings, and I have the right to my choices"

Instead of: "I'm causing problems by not meeting their standards" Try: "Their standards are their preference, not objective requirements"

Instead of: "I should be able to prevent these conflicts" Try: "Conflict is normal when people have different approaches to life"

Managing trauma responses and hypervigilance

Living with constant criticism, optimization pressure, and unpredictable perfectionist episodes can create trauma-like responses in partners, even when the OCPD individual isn't intentionally abusive or harmful.

Hypervigilance, emotional numbing, anxiety about making mistakes, and other trauma responses are normal reactions to chronic stress and emotional unpredictability. Understanding and managing these responses is crucial for maintaining your mental health.

Recognizing trauma responses in OCPD relationships:

Hypervigilance involves constant monitoring of your partner's mood, stress level, and potential triggers to prevent criticism or perfectionist episodes. You may find yourself always alert to environmental factors that might create tension.

Emotional numbing occurs when you shut down your emotional responses to protect yourself from constant criticism or correction. You may feel disconnected from your feelings or unable to access joy, excitement, or other positive emotions.

Anxiety about mistakes develops from repeated exposure to criticism and correction. You may become paralyzed by fear of doing things wrong or spend excessive energy trying to anticipate and prevent errors.

People-pleasing compulsions emerge as strategies for avoiding conflict or criticism. You may find yourself constantly adapting your behavior to prevent triggering your partner's perfectionist anxiety.

Identity confusion results from chronic exposure to messages that your natural approaches are inadequate or wrong. You may lose confidence in your judgment and become unclear about your authentic preferences and values.

Sleep and appetite disruption are common when you're living in chronic stress about performance, criticism, and potential conflict. Your nervous system may remain activated even during rest periods.

Trauma-informed self-care strategies:

Nervous system regulation helps calm your body's stress responses through techniques that activate your parasympathetic nervous system.

Deep breathing exercises: Practice 4-7-8 breathing (inhale for 4, hold for 7, exhale for 8) to signal safety to your nervous system.

Progressive muscle relaxation: Systematically tense and release muscle groups to discharge physical tension and stress.

Cold water exposure: Splash cold water on your face or hold ice cubes to activate your vagus nerve and calm hypervigilance.

Gentle movement: Yoga, walking, or stretching helps discharge stress hormones and reconnect you with your body.

Grounding techniques help you return to the present moment when anxiety about potential criticism or conflict overwhelms you.

5-4-3-2-1 technique: Notice 5 things you can see, 4 things you can touch, 3 things you can hear, 2 things you can smell, and 1 thing you can taste.

Physical grounding: Feel your feet on the ground, notice your breathing, or hold a comforting object to anchor yourself in present reality.

Safe space visualization: Imagine a place where you feel completely safe and calm, engaging all your senses to create a mental refuge.

Reality testing helps you distinguish between past trauma responses and present-moment safety:

Ask yourself: "Am I in immediate danger right now?" "What evidence do I have that something bad is about to happen?" "What would I tell a friend in this situation?"

Trauma recovery resources:

Research shows that trauma-informed therapy approaches can be particularly helpful for partners in emotionally challenging relationships (Van der Kolk, 2014). Several therapeutic modalities specifically address trauma responses:

Eye Movement Desensitization and Reprocessing (EMDR) helps process traumatic memories and reduce their emotional impact. While

OCPD relationships may not involve single traumatic events, EMDR can help with accumulated stress and emotional overwhelm.

Somatic therapies focus on how trauma is stored in the body and use body-based techniques to promote healing and regulation. These approaches can be particularly helpful for hypervigilance and chronic tension.

Cognitive-behavioral therapy helps identify and change thought patterns that maintain trauma responses, such as catastrophic thinking about mistakes or assuming responsibility for others' emotions.

Trauma-sensitive yoga combines gentle movement with mindfulness practices specifically designed for people with trauma histories.

Support group therapy provides validation and coping strategies from others who understand the challenges of difficult relationships.

EMDR and somatic approaches for partner trauma

When traditional talk therapy isn't sufficient for healing the trauma responses created by chronic criticism and control, body-based approaches can provide additional healing pathways.

Understanding how trauma is stored:

Trauma responses aren't just mental—they're stored in your nervous system and body. Years of hypervigilance create physical patterns of tension, stress hormone disruption, and nervous system dysregulation that require body-based healing approaches.

Your body may remain in a state of alert even when your mind knows you're safe. Your nervous system may react to minor criticism as if it's a major threat. Your stress responses may be activated by situations that remind your body of previous experiences of feeling overwhelmed or inadequate.

EMDR for relationship trauma:

EMDR helps process traumatic memories by engaging both sides of the brain while recalling distressing experiences. For OCPD relationship trauma, this might involve processing:

Specific incidents of harsh criticism or humiliation about your approaches or decisions.

Accumulated stress from years of feeling like you can't do anything right.

Anxiety and hypervigilance that developed from living with unpredictable perfectionist episodes.

Loss of identity and confidence that resulted from chronic correction and optimization pressure.

What EMDR treatment involves:

Your therapist will help you identify specific memories or experiences that continue to trigger intense emotional responses. These might be particular conflicts, moments of feeling overwhelmed by criticism, or situations where you felt completely inadequate.

During EMDR sessions, you'll recall these experiences while engaging in bilateral stimulation (usually eye movements, but sometimes tapping or audio tones). This process helps your brain reprocess traumatic memories so they feel less overwhelming and emotionally charged.

Many people report that after EMDR, memories that used to trigger intense shame, anxiety, or helplessness feel more like neutral historical events. The memories remain, but their emotional impact is significantly reduced.

Somatic approaches for nervous system healing:

Somatic therapies recognize that trauma creates changes in how your nervous system responds to stress and relationships. These approaches use body awareness and gentle movement to help restore natural regulation patterns.

Somatic Experiencing focuses on helping your nervous system complete stress responses that may have become stuck or chronic. This might involve learning to notice early signs of activation and practicing techniques for returning to calm states.

Trauma-Sensitive Yoga combines gentle movement with mindfulness practices specifically designed for people with trauma histories. These classes emphasize choice, consent, and internal awareness rather than achieving specific poses.

Body-based mindfulness practices help you reconnect with your body's wisdom and natural regulation abilities. This might include practices like body scanning, mindful breathing, or gentle movement that feels nourishing rather than demanding.

Polyvagal-informed therapies work with your autonomic nervous system to strengthen your capacity for social connection and emotional regulation. These approaches help you develop resilience and flexibility in your stress responses.

Creating daily practices for emotional resilience

Emotional safety in challenging relationships requires consistent, daily practices that build your resilience and maintain your psychological wellbeing over time.

Morning emotional preparation:

Intention setting helps you start each day connected to your values and priorities rather than immediately reacting to external demands or moods.

Spend a few minutes considering: "What kind of person do I want to be today?" "How do I want to respond to challenges?" "What matters most to me today?"

Emotional inventory involves checking in with your current emotional state and any particular needs or vulnerabilities you're aware of.

Ask yourself: "How am I feeling this morning?" "What do I need to take care of myself today?" "Are there any situations I need to prepare for emotionally?"

Affirmation practice provides internal validation and strength that doesn't depend on external circumstances.

Choose affirmations that specifically counter the messages you receive in your relationship: "I am capable and competent," "My feelings and needs matter," "I deserve respect and kindness," "I can handle whatever comes today."

Midday emotional maintenance:

Stress discharge helps prevent accumulation of tension and overwhelm throughout the day.

Take brief breaks to breathe deeply, step outside, stretch, or do whatever helps you release stress before it becomes overwhelming.

Reality checking helps you maintain perspective when criticism or perfectionist pressure distorts your thinking.

Ask yourself: "What's actually true about this situation?" "Am I catastrophizing?" "What would I tell a friend in this situation?" "What evidence do I have for my current thoughts?"

Boundary reinforcement reminds you of your limits and helps you maintain them throughout daily interactions.

Practice phrases like: "I'm not responsible for managing their emotions," "I can care without caretaking," "Their anxiety doesn't have to become my anxiety," "I can listen without agreeing."

Evening emotional processing:

Acknowledgment practice involves recognizing what you handled well during the day, regardless of whether outcomes were optimal.

Notice moments when you maintained your boundaries, expressed your authentic self, made decisions based on your values, or cared for your emotional wellbeing.

Emotional release provides space for processing difficult feelings without judgment or the need to fix them immediately.

Allow yourself to feel frustrated, sad, angry, or overwhelmed without trying to change these emotions. Sometimes just acknowledging them reduces their intensity.

Gratitude practice helps maintain perspective by noting positive aspects of your life, relationships, and personal growth.

This isn't about minimizing problems or practicing toxic positivity—it's about maintaining awareness of what's working alongside what's challenging.

Restoration activities help you reconnect with yourself and replenish your emotional resources.

Engage in activities that feel nourishing rather than demanding: reading, listening to music, taking baths, calling supportive friends, or pursuing hobbies that bring you joy.

Building support networks for emotional safety

Creating emotional safety often requires developing relationships and resources outside your primary partnership that provide validation, perspective, and practical support.

Professional support systems:

Individual therapy with someone who understands personality disorders and relationship trauma can provide crucial guidance and validation for your experiences.

Support groups for partners of people with personality disorders offer connection with others who understand your specific challenges.

Couples therapy may be helpful if your partner is willing to participate and the therapist understands OCPD dynamics.

Psychiatric support can be valuable if you're experiencing depression, anxiety, or other mental health symptoms related to your relationship stress.

Personal support systems:

Trusted friends who provide emotional support and reality-checking when you're questioning your perceptions or experiences.

Family members who knew you before your relationship and can remind you of your strengths and authentic self.

Spiritual or philosophical communities that provide meaning, connection, and perspective on life's challenges.

Interest-based communities through hobbies, classes, or volunteer work that connect you with others who share your values and interests.

Professional networks that support your career growth and remind you of your competence and capabilities.

Online communities for partners of people with OCPD or other personality disorders can provide 24/7 access to understanding and support.

Crisis support resources:

Crisis hotlines provide immediate support during emotional overwhelm or thoughts of self-harm.

Emergency therapy services offer urgent mental health support when your regular resources aren't available.

Trusted friends or family members who you can call during difficult moments for perspective and emotional support.

Safe spaces where you can go when you need to physically remove yourself from overwhelming situations.

Long-term emotional safety planning

Creating sustainable emotional safety requires long-term planning and regular assessment of your strategies and resources.

Safety assessment questions:

Physical safety: Do you feel physically safe in your relationship? Are there any concerns about escalation to physical intimidation or violence?

Emotional safety: Can you express your authentic self without fear of harsh criticism or punishment? Do you feel free to have emotions without being told they're wrong or unreasonable?

Social safety: Are you able to maintain friendships and family relationships? Do you feel comfortable seeking support from others?

Financial safety: Do you have access to money and resources for your own needs? Are you able to make financial decisions within reasonable parameters?

Professional safety: Can you pursue career goals and professional development? Is your partner supportive of your ambitions and achievements?

Parental safety: If you have children, are they protected from inappropriate criticism and impossible standards? Are you able to parent according to your values?

Safety improvement strategies:

Individual therapy to develop coping skills and process relationship trauma

Financial planning to ensure you have resources for independence if needed

Legal consultation if you have concerns about safety or future security

Support network development to reduce isolation and build perspective

Crisis planning so you know what to do during emergencies or overwhelming situations

Documentation of concerning incidents in case professional intervention becomes necessary

Regular safety reviews help you assess whether your current strategies are adequate and what adjustments might be needed.

Monthly questions to consider:

- How effective are my current emotional safety strategies?
- What situations or interactions feel most dangerous to my wellbeing?
- Where do I need additional support or resources?
- Are my boundaries protecting me adequately?
- Do I feel hopeful about my future safety and wellbeing?

Creating emotional safety in an unsafe relationship is challenging work that requires consistency, courage, and often professional support. But it's absolutely possible to develop psychological protection that allows you to function, grow, and maintain hope even in difficult circumstances.

Psychological protection strategies for ongoing exposure

The techniques in this chapter acknowledge that not everyone can or should immediately leave challenging relationships. Sometimes you need time to build resources, protect children, or work on relationship improvement. Sometimes leaving isn't practical or desirable despite ongoing challenges.

In these situations, creating internal emotional safety becomes a crucial life skill. The strategies outlined here help you maintain your psychological wellbeing while navigating ongoing exposure to criticism, perfectionism, and control.

Most importantly, these approaches recognize that your emotional safety matters regardless of your partner's intentions or your relationship's future. You deserve to feel psychologically safe and emotionally stable, and developing these skills serves you regardless of whether your relationship improves, remains stable, or eventually ends.

Your emotional wellbeing is not dependent on your partner's capacity for empathy, flexibility, or change. While those qualities would certainly make your life easier, your psychological safety can be developed and maintained through your own efforts and with appropriate support.

The internal sanctuary you create through these practices becomes a resource you can access throughout your life, providing stability and resilience that no external circumstances can take away from you.

Chapter 13: The parallel life strategy

thriving despite their limitations

When Marcus realized his wife Elena would never share his love of spontaneous weekend adventures, he faced a choice. He could give up the hiking, photography, and exploration that energized him, spend years trying to convince Elena to appreciate unplanned activities, or find a way to pursue these interests while maintaining his marriage.

Marcus chose a fourth option: building what he came to call his "parallel life"—a rich network of experiences, relationships, and pursuits that existed alongside his marriage but didn't require Elena's participation or approval.

Every other Saturday, Marcus joined a hiking group that welcomed his love of discovering new trails without extensive research. He developed friendships with people who enjoyed spontaneous photography expeditions and last-minute dinner invitations. He pursued volunteer work that satisfied his desire to make a difference without requiring Elena's optimization of his charitable choices.

Elena was initially concerned about Marcus's independent activities. "Don't you think that time would be better spent on home projects or family activities?" she asked. But Marcus had learned to appreciate Elena's strengths while protecting his own interests.

"Your organizational skills make our home life run smoothly, and these activities keep me energized and happy," he explained. "Both contribute to our marriage, just in different ways."

Five years later, Marcus describes himself as happier and more fulfilled than he's been in years. His marriage provides stability, financial partnership, and Elena's considerable strengths in planning and organization. His parallel life provides adventure, creativity, and relationships that accept his spontaneous nature.

Most importantly, Marcus has stopped waiting for Elena to become someone different. He's learned to thrive within the constraints of her OCPD while building a life that honors his authentic needs and interests.

Understanding the parallel life strategy

The parallel life approach isn't about secretly rebelling against your partner or building a separate life as preparation for leaving. It's about recognizing that one person cannot and should not be expected to meet all your needs for connection, adventure, intellectual stimulation, or personal growth.

This is particularly important in OCPD relationships because your partner's need for control, optimization, and predictability may create limitations on shared experiences, social connections, or spontaneous activities. Instead of sacrificing these aspects of yourself, you can develop them independently while maintaining your primary relationship.

Key principles of healthy parallel life development:

Complementary rather than competitive: Your independent activities should enhance rather than threaten your primary relationship. They fill gaps in your needs that your partner cannot or will not address, allowing you to bring more satisfaction and less resentment to your marriage.

Transparent rather than secretive: While you don't need your partner's permission for independent activities, maintaining transparency about your interests and commitments builds trust and prevents misunderstandings.

Enriching rather than escapist: Parallel life activities should genuinely contribute to your growth, happiness, and sense of fulfillment rather than simply providing escape from relationship difficulties.

Sustainable rather than reactive: Build independent interests based on your authentic needs and values rather than reactive choices designed to prove your autonomy or frustrate your partner.

Boundaried rather than unlimited: Parallel life development respects your commitments to family, finances, and relationship responsibilities while asserting your right to independent growth and connection.

Common parallel life domains:

Social connections that don't require your partner's participation or approval. These might include friendships based on shared interests your partner doesn't understand, professional networking in areas they don't optimize, or community involvement in causes they don't prioritize.

Creative pursuits that satisfy your need for self-expression without subjecting your creativity to optimization or improvement suggestions. Art classes, writing groups, music activities, or crafting projects that you pursue for personal satisfaction rather than measurable outcomes.

Physical activities that align with your preferences for movement, adventure, or fitness without requiring your partner's participation in activities they find inefficient or uninteresting.

Professional development that reflects your career interests and ambitions rather than your partner's analysis of optimal professional choices. This might include networking, skill development, or career exploration in directions they wouldn't recommend.

Intellectual interests that satisfy your curiosity and learning desires in areas your partner doesn't find practical or valuable. Book clubs, lectures, documentaries, or classes that feed your mind without needing to justify their practical application.

Spiritual or philosophical exploration that addresses your need for meaning and connection in ways your partner's practical worldview doesn't accommodate.

Creating fulfilling experiences they can't control

OCPD partners often have strong opinions about optimal approaches to leisure, social activities, and personal development. Their need to research, plan, and optimize experiences can transform spontaneous adventures into extensively analyzed projects.

Building parallel life experiences requires developing activities that exist outside your partner's sphere of control and optimization, allowing you to reconnect with your natural approaches to fun, learning, and adventure.

Strategies for autonomous experience creation:

Time boundaries protect space for independent activities by establishing regular commitments that don't require negotiation or justification. Join groups that meet weekly, sign up for classes with fixed schedules, or volunteer for organizations that depend on your consistent participation.

Having established commitments makes it easier to maintain independent time without needing to justify each individual choice. Your partner can adapt to "Tuesday evenings are my art class" more easily than they can accept "I want to do art tonight instead of organizing the garage."

Interest-based communities provide built-in social support for activities your partner doesn't understand or appreciate. Photography clubs, hiking groups, book clubs, or hobby organizations create environments where your interests are valued and encouraged rather than analyzed for optimization.

Low-stakes experimentation allows you to try new activities without extensive planning or commitment. Drop-in classes, one-time events, or informal meetups let you explore interests without triggering your partner's need to research the optimal version of whatever you're considering.

Skill development in areas that interest you personally, regardless of whether they align with your partner's vision of practical use of time. Learning languages, musical instruments, artistic techniques, or other skills purely for personal satisfaction rather than measurable outcomes.

Adventure planning that accommodates your spontaneity preferences while respecting your partner's need for security. This might mean joining groups that handle logistics for activities, choosing adventures with built-in safety measures, or planning spontaneous activities within structured time boundaries.

Examples of autonomous experiences:

Sarah's creative parallel life: Sarah joined a pottery studio that offered open studio time alongside structured classes. She could work on projects at her own pace, experiment with techniques that interested her, and connect with other artists without needing to justify her time investment or creative choices to her efficiency-focused husband.

Michael's adventure parallel life: Michael started participating in organized hiking and camping groups that handled safety planning and logistics while preserving opportunities for exploration and discovery. His wife appreciated that these were structured, safe activities while Michael satisfied his need for outdoor adventure.

Jennifer's intellectual parallel life: Jennifer joined multiple book clubs and started attending university lectures open to the public. These activities fed her love of learning and discussion without requiring her husband's participation in topics he found impractical or inefficient.

David's social parallel life: David reconnected with college friends who shared his sense of humor and interest in spontaneous social activities. Their monthly gatherings provided social connection that didn't require optimization or extensive planning.

Tom's service parallel life: Tom began volunteering for organizations that matched his values and interests, providing meaningful work and social connection independent of his partner's opinions about optimal charitable giving or community involvement.

Building chosen family and support systems

OCPD partners may have limited social circles or strong opinions about optimal friendship choices, potentially isolating you from connections that provide emotional support, perspective, and validation.

Building chosen family—relationships that provide emotional support and acceptance—becomes crucial for maintaining your mental health and sense of self in challenging primary relationships.

Understanding chosen family:

Chosen family consists of people who provide emotional support, understanding, and acceptance that you may not receive consistently in your primary relationship. These relationships fill gaps in emotional safety, validation, and encouragement.

Unlike biological family, chosen family is based on mutual care, respect, and emotional connection rather than obligation or circumstance. These relationships develop because people genuinely appreciate and support each other.

Types of chosen family relationships:

Mentor relationships with people who guide your personal or professional development and believe in your potential. These might be former teachers, colleagues, or community members who provide encouragement and wisdom.

Peer support relationships with people facing similar life challenges who understand your experiences without extensive explanation.

Support groups, online communities, or friendships with others in difficult relationships can provide crucial validation.

Authentic friendships with people who appreciate your genuine personality and support your authentic interests. These friends enjoy your company for who you are rather than expecting you to meet specific standards or roles.

Intergenerational relationships that provide different perspectives on life challenges. Older mentors or younger friends can offer wisdom or fresh viewpoints that help you maintain perspective on your situation.

Professional support relationships with therapists, counselors, or coaches who provide objective guidance and emotional support. These relationships offer professional expertise combined with personal care for your wellbeing.

Community connections through shared interests, values, or service that provide belonging and purpose beyond your primary relationship. Religious communities, volunteer organizations, or hobby groups can offer acceptance and connection.

Building chosen family strategically:

Identify relationship needs that aren't being met in your primary partnership. Do you need emotional validation, intellectual stimulation, creative support, adventure companionship, or practical assistance?

Seek communities that naturally include people who might meet these needs. Classes, volunteer organizations, professional associations, or hobby groups often contain potential chosen family members.

Invest in relationships gradually by showing genuine interest in others' lives, offering support when appropriate, and sharing increasingly personal aspects of yourself as trust develops.

Be authentic about who you are and what you need from friendships. Chosen family relationships work best when based on genuine connection rather than performance or adaptation.

Maintain boundaries that protect these relationships from your partner's optimization or criticism. Your chosen family relationships don't need your partner's approval, though they should respect your overall life commitments.

Offer reciprocal support to chosen family members, creating mutual relationships based on care and assistance rather than one-sided emotional dependence.

Pursuing dreams despite their disapproval

OCPD partners often have strong opinions about practical versus impractical life choices. Their need to optimize outcomes may lead them to discourage dreams, goals, or aspirations that seem inefficient, unlikely to succeed, or different from conventional paths to security and achievement.

Learning to pursue meaningful goals despite lack of support from your primary relationship is crucial for maintaining your sense of purpose and personal growth.

Understanding dream suppression in OCPD relationships:

OCPD partners typically analyze goals and dreams through practical filters: Will this make money? Is success likely? Is this an efficient use of time and resources? Are there better alternatives that produce superior outcomes?

While practical analysis has value, dreams and aspirations often involve elements that can't be measured through optimization criteria: personal fulfillment, creative expression, service to others, or pursuit of meaning rather than security.

When your dreams don't pass your partner's practical evaluation, you may face subtle or direct discouragement that gradually erodes your motivation and confidence in your own vision for your life.

Common dream suppression patterns:

Practical alternative suggestions: "Instead of trying to write a novel, why don't you take technical writing courses that could lead to freelance income?"

Risk analysis focus: "Starting a small business has a high failure rate. Have you calculated the potential financial impact on our household?"

Opportunity cost emphasis: "The time you spend on art could be invested in advancing your current career for guaranteed returns."

Logistics overwhelm: "If you want to travel, we need to research optimal destinations, create detailed budgets, and plan itineraries that maximize the experience."

Timeline optimization: "If this is really important to you, let's create a five-year plan with measurable milestones to evaluate whether it's worth continuing."

These responses aren't necessarily meant to discourage you, but they can transform exciting dreams into anxiety-provoking projects subject to efficiency analysis and outcome measurement.

Dream pursuit strategies:

Start privately to protect your initial enthusiasm and momentum from premature analysis or optimization. Begin writing, creating, planning, or researching your interests before involving your partner in detailed discussions about practicality.

Find supportive communities of people pursuing similar dreams who can provide encouragement, practical advice, and understanding of the challenges involved. Writing groups, entrepreneur meetups, artist communities, or hobby organizations offer built-in support systems.

Set your own success metrics based on personal satisfaction, growth, and meaning rather than external measures of achievement or financial return. Define success in ways that reflect your values rather than conventional optimization criteria.

Create manageable timelines that allow for experimentation and learning without requiring immediate results or major life changes. Pursue dreams in ways that fit your current responsibilities while building momentum toward larger goals.

Build skills incrementally through classes, workshops, online learning, or practice that doesn't require major time or financial investment. Develop competence gradually while maintaining other life commitments.

Document progress to maintain motivation and provide evidence of growth even when outcomes aren't immediately visible. Keep journals, portfolios, or records of your learning and development.

Connect dreams to practical benefits when discussing them with your partner. Emphasize skills developed, networks built, stress relief provided, or other outcomes they might appreciate while pursuing personally meaningful goals.

Examples of dream pursuit despite disapproval:

Lisa's writing dream: Despite her husband's concerns about the impracticality of fiction writing, Lisa joined a weekly writing group and committed to writing for 30 minutes each morning before work. She focused on the personal satisfaction and creative outlet rather than publication goals, gradually building skills and confidence.

Mark's music dream: Mark's wife couldn't understand his desire to learn guitar at age 45, but Mark found online lessons and practiced with headphones during times when his musical exploration didn't interfere with household routines. He eventually joined a casual jam group that met monthly.

Rachel's travel dream: Rachel's partner wanted to optimize every vacation for maximum value and experience, which overwhelmed Rachel's desire for spontaneous exploration. Rachel started taking solo day trips to nearby cities and eventually joined a travel group that planned adventures she could enjoy without extensive advance research.

James's service dream: James wanted to volunteer for causes he cared about, but his wife analyzed every organization for efficiency and impact. James quietly started volunteering regularly without extensive discussion, allowing his actions to speak louder than debates about optimal charitable giving.

Financial independence planning

One of the most practical barriers to parallel life development is financial dependence that requires your partner's approval for spending on activities, interests, or relationships they don't value.

Building financial independence—even in small amounts—provides freedom to pursue authentic interests and maintain supportive relationships without constant negotiation or justification.

Understanding financial autonomy needs:

Financial independence for parallel life development doesn't require complete separation of finances or preparation for divorce. It means having access to money you can spend on your personal development, relationships, and interests without detailed justification or optimization analysis.

This might involve separate savings accounts, personal spending allocations, or income from side activities that supports your autonomous choices.

Incremental financial independence strategies:

Personal spending agreements establish amounts you can spend independently without discussion or justification. These might be weekly allowances, monthly budgets, or annual allocations that you manage according to your priorities.

Separate savings accounts for personal interests and goals allow you to build resources for activities, classes, travel, or other pursuits without impacting household finances or requiring approval for each expenditure.

Side income development through freelancing, part-time work, or small business activities can provide additional resources for parallel life activities while potentially developing skills or interests you enjoy.

Expense tracking helps you understand your current spending patterns and identify areas where you might redirect resources toward activities that better support your authentic interests.

Cost-effective parallel life choices maximize your autonomy within limited financial resources:

Free or low-cost activities: Library programs, community events, hiking groups, volunteer organizations, or online learning that provide enrichment without significant expense.

Skill bartering: Exchange services with others to access classes, coaching, or activities without cash investment. Offer your professional skills in exchange for learning opportunities.

Group activities: Join clubs or organizations that share costs for activities, making expensive interests like travel, dining, or entertainment more affordable.

Gradual investment: Build involvement in expensive hobbies or interests slowly, purchasing equipment or paying fees incrementally rather than requiring large upfront investments.

Parallel Life Design Template

This template helps you systematically develop a parallel life that supports your authentic needs while respecting your relationship and family commitments.

Step 1: Needs Assessment

Unmet needs in your primary relationship:

- Emotional support and validation
- Intellectual stimulation and learning
- Creative expression and artistic activities
- Physical adventure and spontaneous activities
- Social connection and friendship
- Professional development and career growth
- Spiritual or philosophical exploration
- Community service and meaningful contribution

Current relationship strengths to preserve:

- Financial stability and security
- Practical support and household management
- Family connections and parenting partnership
- Shared goals and long-term planning
- Professional or social status benefits
- Geographic stability and community connections

Step 2: Parallel Life Vision

Activities I want to pursue independently: Personal interests: _____ Creative pursuits: _____ Physical activities: _____ Learning goals: _____

Social connections: _____ Professional development: _____ Service opportunities: _____

Relationships I want to develop: Mentor relationships: _____ Peer friendships: _____ Professional networks: _____ Community connections: _____ Online communities: _____

Experiences I want to create: Travel and adventure: _____ Cultural activities: _____ Educational experiences: _____ Creative projects: _____ Social events: _____

Step 3: Resource Planning

Time allocation: Daily time available: _____ Weekly time commitments: _____ Monthly activities: _____ Annual goals: _____

Financial resources: Monthly personal spending budget: _____ Annual activity fund: _____ Potential side income sources: _____ Cost-saving strategies: _____

Logistical considerations: Transportation needs: _____ Childcare requirements: _____ Schedule coordination: _____ Equipment or supplies needed: _____

Step 4: Implementation Strategy

First month goals: Activities to start: _____ People to contact: _____ Resources to research: _____ Commitments to make: _____

Three-month goals: Regular activities to establish: _____ Relationships to develop: _____ Skills to build: _____ Experiences to create: _____

One-year vision: Established routines: _____
Developed relationships: _____ Achieved goals:
_____ Overall life satisfaction improvements:
_____

Step 5: Integration Planning

Communication with partner: Information to share:
_____ Boundaries to maintain: _____
Benefits to emphasize: _____ Concerns to address:
_____

Family impact management: Children's needs consideration:
_____ Household responsibility balance:
_____ Schedule coordination: _____
Quality time preservation: _____

Relationship enhancement: How parallel life supports marriage:
_____ Reduced pressure on partner: _____
Increased personal satisfaction: _____ Improved
individual contribution to partnership: _____

Managing partner resistance to parallel life development

Your OCPD partner may initially resist your parallel life
development, viewing it as inefficient use of time, resources, or
energy that could be better optimized for household or family
benefits.

Understanding and preparing for this resistance helps you maintain
your parallel life development while addressing your partner's
concerns constructively.

Common forms of resistance:

Time optimization concerns: "Don't you think that time would be
better spent on home projects, career development, or family
activities?"

Financial efficiency questions: "Is this really the best use of our discretionary income? Have you researched more cost-effective alternatives?"

Social relationship analysis: "These friends don't seem to share our values or priorities. Are these the best social connections for you?"

Activity evaluation: "Have you considered whether this hobby actually contributes to your personal development or if it's just entertainment?"

Priority questioning: "With everything else we need to accomplish, is this really where you want to focus your energy?"

Outcome measurement: "What specific benefits are you getting from these activities? How do you know they're worth the time investment?"

Strategies for managing resistance:

Frame benefits in terms your partner values such as stress reduction that improves your household contribution, skills development that enhances your capabilities, or social connections that provide practical benefits.

"This art class helps me manage stress more effectively, which makes me more patient and present with the family."

"The hiking group keeps me physically fit without requiring expensive gym memberships or equipment."

"These friendships provide emotional support that helps me be a better partner to you."

Emphasize the complementary nature of your parallel life activities rather than positioning them as alternatives to your relationship.

"Your organizational skills handle our household efficiency perfectly. These activities handle my need for creative expression, so I'm not expecting you to fill that role."

"You're excellent at financial planning and practical decisions. This volunteer work satisfies my need to contribute to causes I care about, which makes me more satisfied overall."

Set clear boundaries about activities that are yours to manage independently while acknowledging your partner's right to their concerns.

"I understand you have questions about the practical value of this activity. I'm choosing to pursue it because it fulfills important personal needs for me."

"I appreciate your concern about time management. I've planned these activities so they don't interfere with my household responsibilities or our shared commitments."

Demonstrate rather than argue the benefits of your parallel life activities through consistent positive changes in your mood, energy, and contribution to your relationship.

Let your increased happiness, reduced resentment, and enhanced life satisfaction speak for themselves rather than engaging in lengthy debates about the value of your choices.

Maintain transparency without seeking permission by keeping your partner informed about your activities while making it clear that you're not asking for approval.

"I wanted to let you know I've joined a book club that meets the first Thursday of each month. I'll arrange my schedule so it doesn't conflict with family activities."

"I'm starting volunteer work at the community center on Saturday mornings. I think you'll appreciate having quiet time for your projects while I'm contributing to something meaningful."

Sustaining parallel life over time

Building a parallel life isn't a one-time project—it requires ongoing attention, adjustment, and protection to maintain these important aspects of yourself while managing relationship and family responsibilities.

Long-term sustainability strategies:

Regular assessment of whether your parallel life activities continue to serve your authentic needs rather than becoming obligations or escapes from relationship problems.

Ask yourself quarterly: "Are these activities still energizing me?" "Do they reflect who I am becoming rather than just who I used to be?" "Am I growing through these experiences or just maintaining them out of habit?"

Evolution and adaptation allows your parallel life to change as your needs, interests, and circumstances develop. Be willing to let go of activities that no longer serve you and explore new interests that emerge.

Integration opportunities help you find ways for your parallel life experiences to enrich your primary relationship when possible, while maintaining independence when integration isn't feasible.

You might share skills you've learned, apply insights from your independent activities to household challenges, or invite your partner to occasionally participate in activities they find interesting.

Boundary maintenance protects your parallel life from being optimized, improved, or taken over by your partner's need for control while remaining open to genuine input and concern.

Resource management ensures that your independent activities remain financially and logistically sustainable within your overall life commitments.

Community building within your parallel life creates support systems that help maintain these activities even when your primary relationship goes through difficult periods.

The balance between independence and integration

The goal of parallel life development isn't to create complete separation from your partner or to build a life that competes with your marriage. It's to ensure that important aspects of yourself have space to exist and grow, which ultimately benefits your primary relationship by reducing pressure on your partner to meet all your needs.

Healthy integration principles:

Shared appreciation without shared participation allows you to value what your partner brings to your life while maintaining independent sources of fulfillment.

Mutual support for each other's growth and interests, even when you don't fully understand or participate in those areas.

Reduced expectations on your primary relationship to provide everything you need for happiness and fulfillment.

Enhanced contribution to your partnership from the energy, skills, and satisfaction you gain through independent activities.

Maintained commitment to your shared goals, responsibilities, and family obligations while pursuing individual growth.

The parallel life strategy recognizes that healthy relationships involve interdependence rather than total merger. You can love your partner deeply while acknowledging that they cannot and should not be expected to fulfill every aspect of your human need for connection, growth, and meaning.

How to live fully regardless of partner's constraints

The parallel life strategy outlined in this chapter provides a framework for maintaining your authentic self and pursuing meaningful experiences even when your partner's limitations create constraints on shared activities and goals.

This approach respects your commitment to your relationship while refusing to sacrifice essential aspects of who you are. It acknowledges that OCPD partners have genuine limitations in their ability to appreciate spontaneity, tolerate imperfection, or support activities they consider inefficient, while asserting that these limitations don't have to define the boundaries of your entire life.

Most importantly, the parallel life strategy reduces pressure on your relationship by ensuring that your partner isn't solely responsible for your happiness, fulfillment, and personal growth. This can actually strengthen your primary relationship by allowing both of you to contribute your genuine strengths while having your other needs met through appropriate sources.

Building a parallel life requires courage, planning, and consistent effort, but it offers the possibility of thriving as a complete person rather than simply surviving as an adapted version of yourself. You deserve to experience joy, growth, connection, and meaning in your life, and these experiences can coexist with your commitment to a challenging but valuable primary relationship.

Your parallel life becomes a testament to your resilience, creativity, and refusal to be limited by circumstances beyond your control. It demonstrates that you can love someone deeply while still honoring the fullness of who you are and who you're meant to become.

Chapter 14: If you leave the OCPD divorce survival guide

The decision to leave had been building in Catherine's mind for two years before she finally spoke the words aloud. Her marriage to Robert wasn't abusive in the traditional sense—he'd never threatened her or deliberately tried to harm her. But living with his relentless need to optimize every aspect of their shared life had slowly eroded her sense of self until she felt like a supporting character in someone else's perfectly organized existence.

The breaking point came during their daughter's eighth birthday party. Catherine had spent weeks planning what she thought would be a fun, relaxed celebration with pizza, games, and a dozen neighborhood kids. But Robert couldn't resist improving the event. He reorganized the activities for better flow, optimized the food timing, and provided detailed feedback to Catherine about more efficient party management—all while their daughter watched her mother's excitement deflate under the weight of constant correction.

That night, after the guests had gone home and their daughter was asleep, Catherine found herself staring at Robert as he created a detailed post-event analysis of what could be improved for next year's party. In that moment, she realized she didn't want there to be a next year of this dynamic.

"I can't do this anymore," she said quietly.

Robert looked up from his notes, genuinely confused. "Do what? The party was quite successful once we addressed the logistical issues."

Catherine's heart broke a little as she recognized that Robert truly couldn't see the problem. His optimization of their daughter's party felt helpful and necessary to him. He had no awareness that his improvements had transformed a joyful celebration into an efficiency exercise that left Catherine feeling criticized and their daughter sensing the tension.

"I need to leave," Catherine said. "I need space to find out who I am when I'm not being improved."

This conversation began Catherine's journey through what she now calls "OCPD divorce"—a separation process that required navigating Robert's need to optimize the ending of their marriage, protect their daughter from impossible standards during an already difficult transition, and rebuild her identity while managing practical challenges she'd never handled independently.

Catherine's story illustrates the unique challenges of ending relationships with OCPD partners, who often approach divorce with the same perfectionist intensity they applied to the marriage itself.

Legal strategies for high-conflict divorce

OCPD individuals often approach divorce as a project to be optimized, researched extensively, and managed according to their standards for thorough preparation and superior outcomes. This can create unique legal challenges that require specific strategies to protect your interests and emotional wellbeing.

Understanding OCPD behavior in legal proceedings:

Excessive documentation becomes a tool for proving their position and demonstrating the inadequacy of your approaches to marriage, parenting, or household management. Your partner may compile extensive records of your perceived failures, mistakes, or suboptimal choices.

Micro-management of legal process may involve your partner researching family law extensively, questioning attorney strategies, and insisting on approaches they believe are more thorough or effective than standard legal procedures.

Perfectionist settlement demands can make negotiation difficult when your partner believes they've calculated the objectively fair division of assets and won't accept alternatives that seem inferior to their analysis.

Control through process may manifest as insistence on extensive mediation, detailed documentation of every decision, or refusal to agree to settlements that don't meet their standards for completeness and optimization.

Parenting standard disputes often become central issues when your partner believes their approaches to childcare, education, and development are objectively superior and should govern custody arrangements.

Legal strategies for managing OCPD opposition:

Choose experienced attorneys who understand personality disorders and high-conflict divorce. Look for lawyers who have handled controlling or perfectionist spouses and know how to protect you from manipulation or intimidation through the legal process.

Questions to ask potential attorneys: "Have you handled divorces involving perfectionist or controlling spouses?" "How do you manage cases where one party micro-manages the legal process?" "What strategies do you use when opponents are excessively focused on documentation and detail?" "How do you protect clients from being overwhelmed by their spouse's legal research and demands?"

Document strategically rather than trying to match your partner's extensive record-keeping. Focus on incidents that demonstrate pattern of controlling behavior, impact on your mental health, or effects on children rather than trying to document every disagreement.

Keep records of:

- Incidents where your partner's perfectionist demands affected your mental health

242

- Examples of children becoming anxious or upset due to impossible standards

- Financial control or restrictions on your independence

- Social isolation or discouragement of your support systems

- Escalating criticism or emotional abuse disguised as helpful improvement

Set clear boundaries with your attorney about what level of detail and optimization you're willing to engage in. Don't let your partner's thoroughness pressure you into unnecessarily complicated legal strategies.

"I want a fair settlement, but I'm not interested in fighting over every detail or proving who had better approaches during our marriage."

"My priority is protecting the children and achieving a workable agreement, not optimizing every aspect of asset division."

Use structured negotiation approaches like mediation or collaborative divorce that provide neutral frameworks for decision-making and reduce opportunities for one party to dominate through superior preparation or analysis.

Protect your privacy by limiting the amount of personal information shared during discovery. OCPD partners may use legal proceedings as opportunities to analyze and critique your choices in ways that feel invasive and emotionally harmful.

Focus on children's needs rather than getting drawn into debates about whose parenting standards are superior. Keep discussions centered on practical arrangements that serve children's wellbeing rather than proving parenting competence.

Documentation strategies for emotional abuse

While OCPD relationships may not involve physical violence or obvious emotional abuse, the cumulative effect of constant criticism, control, and impossible standards can be psychologically harmful. Documenting this impact can be important for custody decisions and spousal support considerations.

Types of documentation to maintain:

Pattern documentation shows recurring behaviors rather than isolated incidents. OCPD impact is often cumulative rather than based on single dramatic events.

Keep records of:

- Repeated criticism or correction of your methods and choices
- Instances where your partner took over tasks you were handling adequately
- Times when your partner's standards created anxiety or distress for you or your children
- Examples of social isolation or discouragement of your independent relationships
- Financial control or restrictions on your decision-making authority

Impact documentation records how your partner's behavior affected your mental health, self-esteem, and functioning.

Document:

- Anxiety, depression, or other mental health symptoms that developed or worsened during your marriage
- Loss of confidence in areas where you previously felt competent
- Changes in your social relationships, interests, or goals due to partner's influence
- Physical symptoms of stress related to relationship dynamics

- Professional concerns about your mental health or relationship stress

Children's welfare documentation focuses on how perfectionist pressure affected your children's emotional development and wellbeing.

Record:

- Incidents where children became anxious or upset due to impossible standards

- Changes in children's behavior, confidence, or willingness to try new things

- Examples of children becoming perfectionistic or anxious about making mistakes

- Times when children expressed fear of disappointing the OCPD parent

- Professional concerns from teachers, counselors, or pediatricians about children's stress levels

Communication documentation preserves examples of your partner's communication patterns that demonstrate controlling or critical behavior.

Save:

- Text messages or emails that show excessive criticism or micromanagement

- Examples of your partner researching and correcting your choices

- Communications that demonstrate attempts to control your behavior or decisions

- Messages that show dismissal of your feelings or concerns

- Evidence of your partner preventing or discouraging your independence

Professional documentation includes records from therapists, counselors, or other professionals who observed the relationship dynamics or their effects.

Collect:

- Therapy notes or reports that document relationship stress or emotional abuse

- Medical records showing stress-related symptoms or mental health impacts

- School records indicating children's anxiety or behavioral changes

- Professional recommendations for individual therapy, couples counseling, or separation

Documentation best practices:

Date and time all entries consistently to establish patterns and timelines.

Be factual rather than emotional in your descriptions. Focus on observable behaviors and their effects rather than interpretations or judgments about your partner's motivations.

Include context about circumstances surrounding incidents to help others understand the cumulative impact of seemingly minor events.

Store securely in locations your partner cannot access, including cloud storage with secure passwords or physical documents in safe locations.

Backup regularly to prevent loss of important evidence due to technical problems or discovery.

Share selectively with your attorney, therapist, or other professionals who need to understand your situation, but avoid sharing with friends or family members who might inadvertently compromise your case.

Co-parenting with an OCPD ex-spouse

Divorce doesn't end the challenges of dealing with OCPD behavior—it often intensifies them as your ex-spouse attempts to optimize the co-parenting process according to their standards. Successful co-parenting requires strategies that protect your children while managing ongoing perfectionist pressure.

Understanding post-divorce OCPD behavior:

Parenting standard enforcement may intensify as your ex-spouse tries to maintain their preferred approaches across two households. They may criticize your parenting methods, attempt to establish superior routines, or insist that children follow their standards even in your home.

Information gathering about your household, parenting choices, and children's activities may increase as your ex-spouse tries to maintain control and oversight of situations they can no longer directly manage.

Optimization of custody arrangements can turn routine scheduling into complex negotiations about what's best for children according to your ex-spouse's analysis of optimal parenting time, activities, and environments.

Third-party involvement may increase as your ex-spouse seeks validation for their parenting approaches through teachers, counselors, pediatricians, or other professionals who can confirm their superior methods.

Communication overwhelm through detailed emails, texts, or calls about every aspect of children's care, activities, and development, often with suggestions for improvements to your approaches.

Effective co-parenting strategies:

Parallel parenting rather than collaborative parenting may work better when your ex-spouse's need for control makes genuine collaboration impossible. This approach minimizes direct interaction while ensuring both parents remain actively involved in children's lives.

Under parallel parenting arrangements:

- Each parent has authority over their own household rules and routines

- Communication focuses on essential information about schedules, health, and school rather than parenting philosophy

- Children experience different approaches in each home without pressure to choose sides

- Parents attend separate school conferences and events when possible to reduce conflict opportunities

Structured communication reduces opportunities for criticism and micromanagement while ensuring necessary information is shared.

Use:

- Email for non-urgent communications with clear subject lines and factual content

- Co-parenting apps that track communications and provide neutral platforms for scheduling

- Brief, fact-based messages that avoid emotional content or justifications for your choices

- Response timeframes that allow you to thoughtfully respond rather than react to criticism or demands

Boundary enforcement protects your household autonomy while respecting your ex-spouse's different approaches in their home.

Maintain:

- Clear rules about what decisions require both parents' input versus individual parent authority

- Boundaries around criticism of your parenting methods or household management

- Limits on information sharing about your personal life, relationships, or activities

- Protection of children from being used as messengers or sources of information about your household

Child protection strategies help your children navigate different household standards without becoming anxious or feeling responsible for managing parental conflict.

Teach children:

- That different families have different rules and both are acceptable

- How to handle criticism or pressure about the other parent's household

- That they're not responsible for making either parent happy or reducing conflict

- Age-appropriate information about why parents have different approaches

- Strategies for managing anxiety about meeting different standards in each home

Professional support utilization provides objective guidance and documentation when co-parenting conflicts affect children's wellbeing.

Consider:

- Family therapy to help children adjust to divorce and different parental approaches

- Individual therapy for children showing signs of anxiety or perfectionist pressure

- Co-parenting counseling when conflicts need neutral mediation

- School counselor involvement when academic or social issues arise from family stress

- Legal consultation when your ex-spouse's behavior significantly impacts children's wellbeing

Post-divorce recovery and dating again

Rebuilding your life after ending an OCPD marriage involves recovering from years of criticism and control while learning to trust your own judgment in future relationships. This process requires patience, professional support, and careful attention to patterns that might lead you into similar relationship dynamics.

Identity reconstruction after OCPD marriage:

Rediscovering your preferences involves reconnecting with choices, interests, and values that were suppressed or criticized during your marriage. You may need to relearn what you actually enjoy, prefer, or value independent of someone else's optimization criteria.

Rebuilding decision-making confidence requires practicing choices without extensive research, analysis, or approval-seeking. Start with low-stakes decisions and gradually work toward more significant choices as your confidence rebuilds.

Developing emotional trust in your own feelings and reactions takes time after years of being told that your emotional responses were unreasonable, oversensitive, or illogical.

Reconnecting with your body and its signals about comfort, attraction, and safety may require attention if you became disconnected from physical sensations during a controlling marriage.

Establishing personal boundaries based on your actual limits and needs rather than adapting to someone else's requirements or expectations.

Recovery timeline expectations:

Months 1-6: Focus on basic stability, practical life management, and processing the grief and relief that often accompany the end of difficult marriages. Don't rush into major decisions about career changes, relocating, or new relationships.

Months 6-12: Begin exploring your authentic interests, rebuilding social connections, and developing confidence in independent decision-making. Consider individual therapy to process relationship trauma and develop healthier patterns.

Year 1-2: Start dating casually if desired, while maintaining focus on your own growth and healing. Be particularly alert to red flags that might indicate controlling or perfectionist tendencies in potential partners.

Years 2+: Consider serious relationships when you feel confident in your ability to maintain your identity, boundaries, and independence while also being genuinely intimate with another person.

Red flags in future relationships:

Having experienced OCPD relationship dynamics, you may be particularly vulnerable to partners with similar controlling or perfectionist tendencies. Watch for early warning signs:

Excessive interest in optimizing your choices, methods, or lifestyle during early dating **Criticism disguised as helpfulness** about your approaches to work, parenting, household management, or personal care **Pressure to conform** to their preferences in areas like appearance, social activities, or life goals **Difficulty accepting "no"**

or attempts to negotiate your boundaries and limits **Analysis of your emotions** or attempts to convince you that your feelings are unreasonable or could be improved **Isolation tactics** such as subtle criticism of your friends, family, or support systems **Financial control** including excessive concern about your spending or attempts to optimize your financial decisions **Information gathering** about your past relationships, daily activities, or personal choices that feels invasive

Healthy relationship development:

Gradual intimacy building allows you to maintain your independence and identity while slowly developing trust and connection with new partners.

Open communication about your past relationship experiences helps potential partners understand your needs and boundaries without requiring detailed explanations of your trauma.

Professional support through continued therapy or counseling helps you process relationship patterns and develop skills for healthy intimacy.

Supportive friendships provide perspective and reality-checking as you navigate new relationship possibilities.

Personal goal maintenance ensures that romantic relationships enhance rather than replace your individual growth and development.

Divorce Planning Checklist

This comprehensive checklist helps ensure you address practical and emotional needs during the divorce process while protecting yourself and your children from additional stress and harm.

Legal preparation:

- [ ] Research and interview experienced family law attorneys

- [ ] Gather financial documents (tax returns, bank statements, investment accounts, retirement plans)

- [ ] Document pattern of controlling or harmful behavior

- [ ] Research state laws regarding asset division, spousal support, and child custody

- [ ] Consider mediation or collaborative divorce options

- [ ] Plan for potential high-conflict legal strategies from your spouse

Financial planning:

- [ ] Open individual bank accounts and credit cards in your name only

- [ ] Establish credit history independent of your spouse if needed

- [ ] Document all marital assets and debts

- [ ] Research costs of independent living (housing, utilities, childcare, insurance)

- [ ] Plan for legal fees and other divorce expenses

- [ ] Consider career changes or increases in work hours if needed for financial independence

Housing preparation:

- [ ] Research housing options within your budget and preferred school districts

- [ ] Plan for moving expenses and security deposits

- [ ] Consider temporary housing if needed during transition

- [ ] Arrange for utilities and services in your name

- [ ] Plan for furniture and household items if leaving marital home

Children's needs:

- [ ] Plan age-appropriate conversations about separation and divorce
- [ ] Research therapy or counseling options for children
- [ ] Consider school counselor involvement for additional support
- [ ] Plan custody and visitation schedules that prioritize children's needs
- [ ] Prepare for potential loyalty conflicts and pressure from OCPD spouse
- [ ] Document any negative impacts of spouse's perfectionism on children

Emotional support:

- [ ] Find individual therapist experienced with personality disorder relationships
- [ ] Connect with support groups for divorce or OCPD partners
- [ ] Strengthen relationships with supportive friends and family
- [ ] Plan self-care strategies for managing stress during divorce process
- [ ] Consider medication consultation if experiencing depression or anxiety

Practical considerations:

- [ ] Update beneficiaries on insurance policies, retirement accounts, and other financial instruments
- [ ] Plan for health insurance coverage after divorce

- [ ] Consider name change decisions and associated paperwork

- [ ] Organize important documents in secure, accessible location

- [ ] Plan communication strategies with ex-spouse that minimize conflict

Safety planning (if needed):

- [ ] Identify safe places to go if you need to leave quickly

- [ ] Keep emergency funds accessible

- [ ] Plan for potential escalation of controlling behavior during divorce

- [ ] Document any threats or intimidation

- [ ] Consider restraining orders if safety concerns develop

Managing children's adjustment to divorce

Children in OCPD households often experience unique challenges during divorce because they may have internalized perfectionist standards and feel responsible for maintaining family harmony. Helping them adjust requires attention to their specific vulnerabilities while providing normal divorce support.

Common child reactions in OCPD divorce:

Perfectionist anxiety may increase as children worry about doing everything right to prevent further family problems or to please both parents.

Loyalty conflicts become particularly intense when the OCPD parent believes their approaches are objectively superior and may directly or indirectly pressure children to agree.

Relief mixed with guilt is common when children feel happier with reduced household tension but feel bad about being glad their parents separated.

Fear of mistakes may intensify as children worry that imperfect behavior will create additional family problems or disappoint either parent.

Caretaking behavior may develop as children try to manage their parents' emotions or take responsibility for family harmony.

Age-appropriate divorce support:

Young children (ages 3-7):

- Simple, concrete explanations: "Mom and Dad are going to live in different houses, but we both love you very much"

- Reassurance about their safety and care: "You'll still see both parents regularly and both homes will take good care of you"

- Permission for different rules: "Different houses have different ways of doing things, and that's okay"

- Extra patience with regression or behavioral changes during adjustment

School age (ages 8-12):

- More detailed but still age-appropriate explanations of why parents are divorcing

- Reassurance that the divorce isn't their fault and nothing they could have done would have prevented it

- Help understanding that parents can have different but equally valid approaches to family life

- Support for their own emotional reactions without pressure to choose sides

Teenagers (ages 13-18):

- Honest discussions about family dynamics while avoiding blame or detailed criticism of either parent

- Respect for their ability to form their own opinions about each parent's strengths and weaknesses

- Support for maintaining relationships with both parents even when they disagree with some approaches

- Help developing their own values and standards rather than automatically adopting either parent's approach

Professional support for children:

Individual therapy can help children process their feelings about divorce while learning healthy coping strategies for managing different household expectations.

Family therapy may help when children are struggling with loyalty conflicts or when communication between family members needs improvement.

School counseling provides additional support and may help teachers understand children's home situation when academic or social problems develop.

Support groups for children of divorce can provide peer connection and normalized experiences of family changes.

Building your new life foundation

Successfully recovering from OCPD divorce requires building a life foundation based on your authentic values, needs, and goals rather than reactive choices designed to prove your independence or competence.

Practical foundation building:

Housing that reflects your authentic preferences and provides emotional safety for you and your children, even if it's smaller or less optimized than your marital home.

Financial management based on your values and priorities rather than someone else's optimization criteria, while maintaining responsibility and stability.

Career development that aligns with your interests and goals rather than external expectations about practical or efficient professional choices.

Social connections that appreciate and support your authentic self rather than expecting you to meet specific standards or roles.

Parenting approach that reflects your values while being appropriate for your children's needs and developmental stages.

Emotional foundation building:

Identity clarity about who you are, what matters to you, and what kind of life you want to create independent of others' opinions or optimization.

Boundary confidence in your ability to maintain your limits and needs even when others disapprove or pressure you to change.

Decision-making trust in your judgment and ability to make choices that serve your wellbeing even when they're not perfect or optimal.

Relationship skills for developing healthy intimacy while maintaining independence and autonomy.

Stress management abilities that help you navigate challenges without becoming overwhelmed or reverting to people-pleasing patterns.

The goal isn't to become someone completely different or to reject everything from your previous life. It's to build a life that honors who you actually are while incorporating the positive lessons and skills you developed during your marriage.

Recovery from OCPD divorce is possible, and many people report feeling happier, more confident, and more authentic after the difficult transition period. With appropriate support, realistic expectations, and commitment to your own healing, you can create a life that feels genuinely yours while maintaining positive relationships with your children and, when possible, cooperative co-parenting with your ex-spouse.

Practical guidance for navigating separation

The strategies in this chapter acknowledge that leaving an OCPD marriage involves unique challenges that standard divorce advice doesn't address. OCPD partners often approach divorce with the same perfectionist intensity they brought to marriage, creating additional stress and complication for an already difficult process.

Understanding these dynamics helps you prepare emotionally and practically for the specific challenges you're likely to face while protecting yourself and your children from additional harm during an already vulnerable time.

Most importantly, this guidance recognizes that choosing to leave doesn't mean you've failed at your marriage or given up too easily. Sometimes the most loving choice—for yourself, your children, and even your spouse—is creating space for everyone to find situations that better match their needs and capabilities.

Your decision to prioritize your mental health and authentic self demonstrates courage and wisdom, not weakness or selfishness. The practical strategies in this chapter help ensure that your transition to independence is as smooth and safe as possible while laying the foundation for a life that truly reflects who you are and what matters most to you.

Chapter 15: The relationship reset—new patterns for lasting change

After eighteen months of individual therapy, couples counseling, and medication that helped manage his perfectionist anxiety, David sat across from his wife Michelle at their kitchen table with a document he'd been working on for weeks. But this wasn't another one of his characteristic optimization projects with detailed analysis and systematic improvements.

This was different. For the first time in their twelve-year marriage, David was acknowledging that his need to control and improve everything had created problems that needed addressing—not through better systems, but through fundamental changes in how they related to each other.

"I've been thinking about what our therapist said about relationship agreements," David began, his voice carrying a vulnerability Michelle hadn't heard before. "I realize I've been trying to optimize our marriage without asking what you actually needed from me."

The document in front of them wasn't a complex contract with subclauses and contingencies. It was a simple one-page agreement outlining how they wanted to handle the recurring issues that had created years of tension: David's need to improve Michelle's methods, Michelle's need for autonomy in her choices, their different approaches to parenting, and their struggles with intimacy when perfectionist anxiety overwhelmed emotional connection.

Michelle looked at the paper with cautious hope. They'd tried to change their patterns before, but those attempts usually involved

David researching better communication techniques or Michelle trying harder to appreciate his helpful suggestions. This felt different—like they were finally addressing the actual problems instead of optimizing around them.

Six months later, David and Michelle describe their relationship as better than it's ever been. Not perfect (a concept they've learned to question), but genuinely satisfying for both of them. They still have different approaches to tasks and decisions, but they've learned to appreciate these differences rather than trying to eliminate them through improvement or adaptation.

Their transformation didn't happen through dramatic personality changes or sudden insights. It happened through structured, consistent work on developing new patterns that honored both David's need for order and Michelle's need for autonomy.

Creating relationship agreements that work with OCPD

Traditional relationship advice often assumes both partners can simply agree to communicate better, be more flexible, or try harder to understand each other's perspectives. But OCPD thinking patterns make these generic approaches ineffective because the fundamental issue isn't lack of effort—it's the way perfectionist brains process information about efficiency, standards, and optimal outcomes.

Effective relationship agreements for OCPD couples must work with these thinking patterns rather than against them, providing structure and clarity that satisfies the OCPD partner's need for systematic approaches while protecting the non-OCPD partner's autonomy and emotional wellbeing.

Understanding why standard relationship approaches fail with OCPD:

"Try to be more flexible" doesn't work because flexibility feels like accepting inferior outcomes when better alternatives are available. OCPD individuals need specific frameworks for when flexibility is appropriate and when standards should be maintained.

"Communicate your feelings better" doesn't work because OCPD partners often interpret emotional expressions as problems to be solved rather than experiences to be understood. They need guidelines for when to listen versus when to problem-solve.

"Compromise more" doesn't work because compromise feels like both people settling for less than optimal outcomes. OCPD individuals need win-win structures where both partners get their core needs met without sacrificing quality.

"Accept each other's differences" doesn't work because OCPD thinking categorizes differences as opportunities for improvement rather than neutral variations. They need frameworks that position differences as complementary strengths rather than problems to be resolved.

Elements of effective OCPD relationship agreements:

Specific behavioral commitments rather than vague promises to "do better" or "try harder." OCPD individuals respond well to clear, measurable actions they can implement consistently.

Instead of: "I'll be more supportive of your choices" Try: "When you're making decisions about social plans, I'll offer input only when you specifically ask for it"

Clear authority divisions that specify who has primary decision-making power in different life areas, reducing the need for ongoing negotiation about whose approach should prevail.

"You handle all social planning and restaurant choices. I handle all financial planning and major purchase research. We consult each other but respect the primary decision-maker's final choice."

Process agreements that outline how you'll handle recurring situations rather than trying to resolve each incident through discussion and compromise.

"When we disagree about household tasks, we'll use the timer method: each person handles the task their way on alternating weeks, and we evaluate results after one month."

Emotional safety protocols that protect both partners' wellbeing when perfectionist anxiety or criticism overwhelm the relationship dynamic.

"When either person feels overwhelmed by optimization pressure, they can call a 'pause' and we'll return to the discussion after a 30-minute break."

Progress tracking systems that appeal to the OCPD partner's need to measure improvements while focusing on relationship satisfaction rather than perfect execution.

"We'll check in weekly about how our agreements are working and make adjustments as needed, celebrating what's improving rather than focusing on what still needs fixing."

Sample relationship agreement framework:

Household Management Agreement:

- Person A has primary authority over: [specific areas]

- Person B has primary authority over: [specific areas]

- Shared decisions require agreement: [major purchases over $X, children's school choices, etc.]

- Input is welcome when requested, not required when not asked

- "Good enough" standards are acceptable in all areas unless safety is involved

Communication Agreement:

- Emotional expressions receive empathy first, problem-solving only when requested

- Criticism of methods is replaced with appreciation of outcomes

- Suggestions are offered as options, not improvements that should be implemented

- Both partners can request discussion breaks when conversations become overwhelming

- We focus on what we want to create together rather than analyzing what's wrong

Parenting Agreement:

- We support each other's different strengths without trying to make approaches identical

- Children benefit from exposure to different perspectives on organization, creativity, and problem-solving

- We present united fronts on major rules while allowing different styles in implementation

- Both parents' approaches are valid; children don't need to choose the "better" way

- We seek professional guidance when our different approaches create confusion for children

Intimacy Agreement:

- Physical affection happens without performance pressure or optimization analysis

- Emotional sharing is appreciated without being immediately improved or solved

- We create regular time for connection that doesn't involve household management or problem-solving

- Both partners can request intimacy (emotional or physical) without being analyzed for efficiency

- We celebrate our connection rather than constantly working to improve it

Intimacy building despite emotional constriction

OCPD individuals often struggle with emotional intimacy because their brains automatically analyze and try to optimize emotional experiences rather than simply allowing them to unfold naturally. This can make partners feel like their emotions are being treated as problems to be solved rather than experiences to be shared and understood.

Building genuine intimacy requires creating space for unanalyzed emotional connection while respecting the OCPD partner's natural tendency toward structure and improvement.

Understanding intimacy challenges in OCPD relationships:

Emotional optimization occurs when the OCPD partner tries to help you feel better by solving whatever created your emotions rather than simply acknowledging and accepting your feelings.

When you're sad about a difficult day, your partner might immediately offer solutions for handling the situation more efficiently next time instead of just providing comfort and understanding.

Performance anxiety develops around emotional expression when you learn that sharing feelings often triggers analysis and improvement suggestions rather than empathy and connection.

You may stop sharing disappointments, frustrations, or even positive emotions if they consistently get redirected toward problem-solving rather than emotional connection.

Vulnerability resistance happens when the OCPD partner struggles to share their own emotions because they're not sure how to express feelings that can't be optimized or improved.

They may have difficulty articulating anxiety, sadness, or uncertainty because these emotions feel like problems that should be solved rather than experiences to be shared.

Physical intimacy pressure can develop when the OCPD partner approaches physical connection with the same goal-oriented focus they apply to other activities, creating performance pressure rather than natural connection.

Spontaneity challenges occur because intimacy often requires unplanned moments of connection that conflict with the OCPD partner's need for structure and predictability.

Strategies for building authentic intimacy:

Create structured space for unstructured connection by scheduling regular time for emotional sharing that has clear boundaries around problem-solving.

"Every Tuesday evening, we spend 30 minutes sharing how we're feeling about our lives, our relationship, and our individual experiences. This is listening time, not fixing time."

Develop empathy-first communication where emotional expressions receive acknowledgment and understanding before any problem-solving is offered.

Practice phrases like: "That sounds really frustrating," "I can see why you'd feel that way," "Thank you for sharing that with me," before moving to "Would you like suggestions, or do you just want me to understand?"

Build appreciation practices that focus on what you value about each other rather than areas for improvement.

Weekly appreciation exchanges where each partner shares three specific things they appreciated about the other person's actions, choices, or qualities during the week.

Create intimacy rituals that don't have performance goals or outcome measures, focusing on connection rather than achievement.

Daily check-ins, weekly walks without phones, monthly date nights with no agenda other than enjoying each other's company, or bedtime conversations about positive moments from the day.

Practice vulnerability in small doses by sharing feelings, concerns, or experiences that don't require solutions, gradually building comfort with emotional expression that doesn't lead to optimization.

Establish physical affection agreements that remove performance pressure and allow natural physical connection to develop without analysis or improvement.

"Physical affection happens for connection and pleasure, not to achieve specific outcomes. We can touch, hug, and be intimate without analyzing whether we're doing it optimally."

The weekly relationship meeting format

Regular relationship meetings provide structure that appeals to OCPD thinking while ensuring that both partners' needs get addressed systematically. These meetings work because they satisfy the OCPD partner's need for organized communication while protecting the non-OCPD partner from constant feedback and optimization pressure.

Why weekly meetings work for OCPD relationships:

Contained optimization gives the OCPD partner a specific time and place for relationship analysis and improvement suggestions, reducing the need for constant feedback throughout the week.

Structured emotional expression provides a safe format for sharing feelings and concerns without triggering immediate problem-solving responses.

Preventive maintenance appeals to the OCPD partner's preference for systematic approaches to maintaining important systems— including relationships.

267

Equal participation ensures both partners' voices are heard and valued rather than allowing the OCPD partner's analytical style to dominate all relationship discussions.

Progress tracking satisfies the OCPD partner's need to see measurable improvement while focusing on positive changes rather than deficit correction.

Weekly meeting structure (45-60 minutes):

Check-in round (10 minutes): Each partner shares their overall emotional and energy state, highlights from the week, and any particular needs or concerns they're aware of. No advice or problem-solving during this segment—just listening and acknowledgment.

Appreciation round (10 minutes): Each partner shares three specific things they appreciated about the other person during the week. Focus on actions, choices, or qualities rather than general compliments. This builds positive momentum before addressing challenges.

Agreement review (10 minutes): Review how your relationship agreements worked during the week. What went well? Where did you struggle? What adjustments might help? Focus on the system rather than blaming individuals for implementation challenges.

Issue resolution (15 minutes maximum): Address one specific issue that needs discussion or problem-solving. Use structured communication: each person gets to share their perspective without interruption, then you work together on solutions. If more time is needed, schedule another conversation rather than extending the meeting.

Planning and coordination (10 minutes): Discuss upcoming schedules, events, decisions, or activities that need coordination. Handle logistics efficiently while making sure both partners' preferences and needs are considered.

Connection time (5-10 minutes): End with positive focus on your relationship: what you're looking forward to together, expressions of care and commitment, or simply enjoying each other's company without any agenda.

Meeting ground rules:

One issue per meeting prevents problem-solving from overwhelming connection and appreciation time.

No surprises means major issues get mentioned ahead of time so both partners can prepare emotionally for difficult discussions.

Equal talking time ensures both partners' perspectives get heard fully before solutions are considered.

Focus on the future emphasizes what you want to create together rather than relitigating past problems or mistakes.

Celebration before criticism builds positive momentum before addressing challenges or areas for improvement.

Solution orientation moves quickly from problem identification to collaborative brainstorming about improvements.

Celebrating small wins and incremental progress

OCPD individuals often struggle to appreciate partial improvements or imperfect progress because their focus on optimization makes "good enough" feel unsatisfying. But relationship change happens gradually, and learning to celebrate incremental progress is crucial for maintaining motivation and momentum.

Why celebration matters for OCPD relationships:

Reinforces positive changes by acknowledging when new behaviors are working, even if they're not perfect or consistent yet.

Counters perfectionist thinking that dismisses improvements as inadequate because they haven't reached optimal levels.

Builds motivation for continued effort by highlighting progress rather than focusing on remaining areas for improvement.

Strengthens emotional connection through shared positive experiences and mutual appreciation.

Creates hopeful perspective by demonstrating that change is possible and worthwhile even when it's gradual.

Types of progress worth celebrating:

Behavioral changes when either partner tries new approaches, even if they don't work perfectly:

- OCPD partner offers input without taking over a task

- Non-OCPD partner expresses needs clearly without apologizing for having preferences

- Both partners use pause techniques during potential conflicts

- Either person acknowledges mistakes without extensive self-criticism

Communication improvements in how you talk to each other about differences, problems, or feelings:

- Listening without immediately offering solutions

- Expressing appreciation alongside requests for change

- Asking for clarification instead of assuming negative motivations

- Sharing emotions without extensive justification

Relationship satisfaction indicators that show your connection is strengthening:

- Enjoying each other's company more often

- Feeling more comfortable being authentic with each other

- Experiencing less daily tension about household management

- Looking forward to time together rather than feeling drained by interaction

Individual growth that benefits the relationship:

- OCPD partner developing tolerance for "good enough" outcomes
- Non-OCPD partner building confidence in their decision-making
- Both partners pursuing individual interests while maintaining connection
- Either person seeking professional support for personal development

Effective celebration strategies:

Specific acknowledgment of what changed and why it mattered: "I really appreciated how you listened to my concerns about the vacation planning without immediately researching better alternatives. That helped me feel heard and valued."

Progress tracking that emphasizes improvement over perfection: "Three months ago, discussions about household organization always became tense. Now we can talk about different approaches without either of us getting defensive."

Future-focused appreciation that builds momentum toward continued growth: "I'm excited about how we're learning to appreciate each other's different strengths instead of trying to make our approaches identical."

Small ritual celebrations that mark progress without creating performance pressure: Special dinners when you successfully navigate a difficult conversation, small gifts to acknowledge effort and growth, or planned activities to celebrate relationship milestones.

Shared reflection on how far you've come and what made the difference: "What do you think helped us handle that disagreement differently this time?" "How does our relationship feel different now compared to six months ago?"

Relationship Reset Contract Template

This template provides a framework for creating written agreements that work with OCPD thinking patterns while protecting both partners' core needs. Customize it based on your specific relationship challenges and goals.

Our Relationship Reset Agreement

Date: _____ **Review Date:** _____

Our shared commitment: We choose to build a relationship that honors both our needs for order and autonomy, appreciating our different strengths while creating harmony and connection.

Section 1: Decision-Making Authority

[Partner A] has primary authority for:

- [ ] Social planning and restaurant choices
- [ ] Children's daily routines and activities
- [ ] Home decorating and organization systems
- [ ] Weekend and vacation activities
- [ ] Gift-giving and holiday planning
- [ ] Other: _____

[Partner B] has primary authority for:

- [ ] Financial planning and major purchases
- [ ] Home maintenance and repairs
- [ ] Career and professional development decisions

- [ ] Technology choices and household systems
- [ ] Insurance and healthcare decisions
- [ ] Other: _____

Shared decisions requiring agreement:

- [ ] Children's education and school choices
- [ ] Major purchases over $_____
- [ ] Moving or housing changes
- [ ] Extended family relationship decisions
- [ ] Health and medical decisions
- [ ] Other: _____

Section 2: Communication Agreements

When sharing emotions or concerns, we agree to:

- Listen first, offer solutions only when requested
- Acknowledge each other's feelings before providing different perspectives
- Use "I" statements about our own experiences rather than "you" statements about the other's behavior
- Take breaks when conversations become overwhelming or heated
- Focus on what we want to create together rather than what's wrong

When offering input or suggestions, we agree to:

- Ask permission before providing advice about the other's methods or choices

- Present suggestions as options rather than improvements that should be implemented

- Accept "no thank you" without extended explanation or persuasion

- Appreciate the other's competence even when their approaches differ from our preferences

- Offer specific help rather than general criticism

Section 3: Household Management

We agree that:

- "Good enough" is acceptable in all areas unless safety is involved

- Different approaches to organization and efficiency are both valid

- Each person's standards apply in their areas of authority

- Help is offered when requested, not automatically provided

- Both partners contribute according to their strengths and availability

When disagreements arise about household tasks, we will:

- Use the "try it your way" approach for one week, then evaluate results

- Focus on outcomes that work for our family rather than optimal methods

- Respect each other's different relationships with mess, order, and efficiency

- Ask for specific support when we need it rather than expecting mind-reading

Section 4: Parenting Partnership

We commit to:

- Supporting each other's different parenting strengths without trying to make our approaches identical

- Presenting united fronts on major rules while allowing different styles in implementation

- Protecting children from adult disagreements about methods and standards

- Seeking professional guidance when our differences create confusion for children

- Celebrating our children's efforts and growth rather than only acknowledging perfect performance

We will not:

- Criticize each other's parenting methods in front of the children

- Use children as messengers or sources of information about the other parent

- Create impossible standards that make children anxious about making mistakes

- Compete about whose approach produces better results

Section 5: Intimacy and Connection

We agree to create regular time for:

- Physical affection without performance pressure or analysis

- Emotional sharing that doesn't require problem-solving

- Fun activities that we both enjoy without optimizing the experience

- Appreciation and gratitude for what we value about each other

- Sexual intimacy based on mutual desire rather than scheduled efficiency

We promise to:

- Accept each other's different needs for social interaction, alone time, and emotional expression
- Share our own feelings and needs without expecting the other to fix them
- Create space for spontaneity and unplanned connection
- Prioritize our relationship health alongside individual goals and family responsibilities

Section 6: Individual Growth Support

We commit to supporting each other's:

- Professional development and career goals
- Individual friendships and social connections
- Personal interests and hobbies
- Mental health and self-care practices
- Spiritual or philosophical exploration

We agree to:

- Maintain our individual identities while building our partnership
- Encourage each other's growth even when it involves approaches we don't fully understand
- Provide emotional support during challenging times without trying to fix everything
- Celebrate each other's achievements and personal victories

Section 7: Review and Adjustment Process

We will:

- Review this agreement monthly during our weekly relationship meetings

- Make adjustments based on what's working and what needs improvement

- Celebrate progress and acknowledge areas where we're still growing

- Seek professional help when we need objective guidance or support

- Recommit to these agreements regularly rather than assuming they'll maintain themselves automatically

Our signatures indicate commitment to working on these agreements with patience, kindness, and genuine effort to create the relationship we both want.

[Partner A]: _____ Date: _____ [Partner B]: _____ Date: _____

Maintaining momentum during setbacks

Even with clear agreements and consistent effort, OCPD relationships will experience setbacks when stress, life changes, or old patterns temporarily overwhelm your new approaches. Maintaining momentum during these difficult periods requires realistic expectations and specific strategies for getting back on track.

Common setback triggers:

High stress periods such as job changes, family illness, financial pressure, or major life transitions can cause both partners to revert to familiar patterns even when those patterns aren't healthy.

Holiday and family events often trigger perfectionist anxiety and control issues, making it difficult to maintain the flexibility and respect you've developed in normal circumstances.

Children's challenges with school, behavior, or development can activate parental anxiety and disagreements about the best approaches to handling problems.

Communication breakdowns when one difficult conversation escalates and damages the trust and goodwill you've been building over time.

External pressures from work, extended family, or community that create additional stress and reduce your capacity for relationship patience and flexibility.

Setback recovery strategies:

Normalize temporary regression rather than viewing setbacks as evidence that your progress wasn't real or sustainable.

"We're having a hard time with our communication agreements right now because we're both stressed about the job situation. This doesn't mean our progress wasn't real—it means we need extra support during difficult periods."

Return to basics by focusing on the most essential agreements rather than trying to maintain perfect execution of all your relationship improvements.

During stressful periods, prioritize emotional safety and respect while allowing flexibility with less critical agreements about household management or decision-making processes.

Seek additional support through therapy, couples counseling, or professional consultation when setbacks persist or create significant relationship damage.

Use repair conversations to acknowledge what went wrong and recommit to your agreements without extensive analysis of why the setback occurred.

"I know we both handled that disagreement in ways that didn't match our communication agreements. Can we start over and try a different approach?"

Focus on learning rather than blame when examining what contributed to temporary regression.

"What was different about this situation that made it harder for us to use our usual strategies? How can we prepare better for similar challenges in the future?"

Long-term relationship sustainability

Building lasting change in OCPD relationships requires understanding that this is ongoing work rather than a problem that gets solved once and remains fixed. Sustainable relationships develop systems for continuous improvement while accepting that perfection isn't the goal.

Sustainability principles:

Progress over perfection acknowledges that relationships involve continuous growth and adjustment rather than achieving an optimal state that requires no further work.

Flexibility within structure provides enough organization to satisfy OCPD needs while allowing adaptation as circumstances and individuals change over time.

Individual growth alongside partnership ensures that both partners continue developing as individuals while building their relationship together.

Professional support integration makes therapy, counseling, or other professional guidance a normal part of relationship maintenance rather than crisis intervention.

Community support systems provide perspective, encouragement, and practical assistance that reduces pressure on the relationship to meet all emotional and social needs.

Annual relationship planning:

Many successful OCPD couples develop yearly planning processes that review relationship satisfaction, adjust agreements as needed, and set goals for continued growth and connection.

Annual review questions:

- What aspects of our relationship are working well and should be maintained?

- Where do we still experience regular tension or dissatisfaction?

- How have we each grown as individuals this year, and how has that affected our partnership?

- What goals do we have for our relationship in the coming year?

- What support or resources would help us continue improving our connection?

Goal setting for relationship development:

- Communication skills we want to develop further

- Areas where we want to build more appreciation and understanding

- Activities or experiences we want to share together

- Individual growth that would benefit our partnership

- Professional support or resources we want to utilize

The relationship reset process outlined in this chapter provides a framework for creating lasting positive change in OCPD relationships. It works because it honors both partners' needs while providing structure that satisfies perfectionist thinking patterns.

Structured approaches to relationship improvement

The strategies in this chapter acknowledge that generic relationship advice doesn't work for OCPD couples because it doesn't account for how perfectionist thinking affects communication, decision-making, and emotional connection. Effective approaches must provide clear structure while protecting autonomy, specific agreements while allowing flexibility, and systematic improvement without performance pressure.

Most importantly, these structured approaches recognize that both partners bring valuable strengths to the relationship. The goal isn't to eliminate OCPD traits or force the non-OCPD partner to adapt completely. The goal is to create agreements that allow both people to contribute their best qualities while having their core needs respected and met.

Relationship reset work requires patience, consistency, and genuine commitment from both partners. But couples who engage in this process often report feeling more connected, appreciated, and hopeful about their future together than they have in years. The structure provides safety for both partners to be authentic while building the skills needed for lasting intimacy and partnership.

Chapter 16: Your emergency toolkit and maintenance plan

The call came at 2:47 AM on a Tuesday. Jennifer's voice was shaky but determined as she whispered into the phone, "I need help. Mark's perfectionist anxiety spiraled tonight over our daughter's school project, and I realized I can't handle another episode like this without a plan."

Her friend Sarah, who'd been through her own OCPD relationship challenges years earlier, recognized the familiar pattern: everything had been going well, the couple had been using their communication techniques successfully, but one unexpected stressor had triggered old patterns of criticism, control, and emotional overwhelm that left both partners feeling defeated.

"Do you remember your emergency protocols?" Sarah asked gently. "The plan we worked out last year for exactly this kind of situation?"

Jennifer felt a wave of relief wash over her. She did have a plan. She'd forgotten about it during the chaos of Mark's escalating anxiety about their daughter's "substandard" poster board presentation, but the emergency toolkit she'd developed was still there, waiting to be used.

By morning, Jennifer had implemented her crisis intervention strategies, reconnected with her support system, and scheduled an emergency session with their couples therapist. What could have become a relationship-damaging spiral became a manageable setback that they recovered from within a week.

The difference wasn't that their relationship had become perfect or that Mark's OCPD symptoms had disappeared. The difference was that Jennifer had prepared for setbacks by developing comprehensive systems for managing crisis situations and maintaining long-term relationship health.

This chapter provides those same systems—practical tools, emergency protocols, and maintenance plans that help you manage both crisis moments and ongoing relationship challenges with confidence and competence.

Crisis intervention protocols

OCPD relationships can experience sudden escalations when perfectionist anxiety overwhelms normal coping strategies, creating intense conflicts that feel devastating and unrecoverable. Having predetermined crisis protocols helps you respond effectively rather than reactively, preventing temporary setbacks from becoming permanent damage.

Recognizing crisis indicators:

Perfectionist anxiety escalation occurs when your partner becomes overwhelmed by inefficiency, mess, or suboptimal outcomes and responds with intense criticism, attempt to control everything, or emotional shutdown.

Warning signs include: rapid-fire improvements suggestions, taking over multiple tasks simultaneously, expressing desperation about "chaos" or "things falling apart," or becoming paralyzed by the impossibility of getting everything right.

Partner emotional overwhelm happens when you feel completely flooded by criticism, corrections, or perfectionist pressure and lose your ability to maintain boundaries or communicate clearly.

Warning signs include: feeling like you can't do anything right, wanting to escape or hide, losing your sense of competence, or feeling angry enough to say things you'll regret later.

Communication breakdown occurs when your usual strategies stop working and conversations escalate into arguments about whose approach is better rather than collaborative problem-solving.

Warning signs include: rehashing old grievances, character attacks rather than behavior discussions, both people becoming defensive simultaneously, or conversations that circle endlessly without resolution.

Family system stress affects everyone when perfectionist pressure creates household tension that impacts children, extended family relationships, or other important connections.

Warning signs include: children becoming anxious or asking if parents are getting divorced, social isolation due to embarrassment about relationship conflicts, or other family members expressing concern about household dynamics.

Immediate crisis interventions:

Physical separation provides space for emotional regulation when interactions are escalating rather than problem-solving.

"I can see we're both overwhelmed right now. I'm going to take a 30-minute break to collect myself, and then we can try this conversation again."

Breathing and grounding techniques help regulate nervous systems that are activated by conflict and perfectionist anxiety.

Practice 4-7-8 breathing (inhale for 4, hold for 7, exhale for 8) or 5-4-3-2-1 grounding (notice 5 things you see, 4 you can touch, 3 you can hear, 2 you can smell, 1 you can taste).

Crisis perspective statements remind both of you that this is a temporary setback rather than evidence of fundamental relationship failure.

"This is anxiety talking, not our normal thinking. We can handle this differently when we're calmer."

"We've gotten through difficult moments before. This feels overwhelming right now, but it's not permanent."

Support system activation connects you with people who can provide immediate emotional support and perspective during crisis moments.

Call trusted friends, family members, or professionals who understand your situation and can offer encouragement and practical guidance.

Safety assessment ensures that crisis situations don't escalate to emotional abuse or threats that require immediate intervention.

If your partner's perfectionist anxiety includes threats, intimidation, or behavior that makes you feel unsafe, prioritize your immediate safety over relationship preservation.

24-hour crisis protocols:

Hour 1: Immediate safety and regulation

- Ensure physical safety for everyone involved
- Implement breathing and grounding techniques
- Create physical space if interactions are escalating
- Activate emergency support contacts if needed

Hours 2-6: Initial stabilization

- Use individual coping strategies rather than trying to fix the relationship crisis immediately
- Engage in self-care activities that help you feel more stable and centered
- Avoid making major decisions about your relationship while emotions are high
- Focus on meeting basic needs (food, rest, comfort) for yourself and any children

Hours 6-12: Perspective recovery

- Begin using cognitive techniques to challenge catastrophic thinking

- Review what triggered the crisis and what factors made it escalate

- Connect with support systems for validation and reality-checking

- Start planning how to approach repair conversations when both people are calmer

Hours 12-24: Repair planning

- Schedule specific time for relationship discussion when both partners are regulated

- Plan what needs to be addressed versus what can be set aside for now

- Identify what support resources you need for moving forward

- Commit to one small step toward repair rather than trying to solve everything immediately

The 30-day relationship rescue plan

When your relationship feels like it's in serious trouble but you want to try intensive improvement before making major decisions about your future, a structured 30-day rescue plan can provide focused effort and clear evaluation criteria.

Understanding when rescue plans are appropriate:

Temporary crisis situations where external stressors have overwhelmed your usual coping strategies but the underlying relationship foundation remains solid.

Recent insight development when one or both partners have gained new understanding about OCPD patterns and are motivated to implement significant changes.

Professional support availability when you have access to therapy, counseling, or other guidance to support intensive relationship work.

Mutual commitment when both partners are genuinely willing to prioritize relationship improvement for a specific time period.

Clear evaluation criteria so you can assess whether intensive efforts are producing meaningful change or whether other decisions need to be considered.

Week 1: Stabilization and commitment

Days 1-2: Crisis de-escalation

- Implement immediate safety and communication protocols
- Agree on basic ground rules for respectful interaction
- Schedule daily check-ins to monitor emotional temperature
- Commit to 30-day intensive improvement effort

Days 3-4: Professional support activation

- Schedule emergency couples therapy session
- Research additional resources (support groups, relationship programs, etc.)
- Individual therapy sessions for any needed mental health support
- Create accountability plan with professional guidance

Days 5-7: Pattern identification

- Review recent conflicts to identify triggers and escalation patterns
- Document what approaches have worked versus what consistently fails

- Identify each person's core relationship needs that must be addressed

- Set specific, measurable goals for the 30-day period

Week 2: Implementation of new strategies

Days 8-10: Communication overhaul

- Practice new communication techniques daily with low-stakes topics

- Implement structured conversation formats for difficult discussions

- Use professional guidance to navigate specific relationship issues

- Focus on listening and understanding rather than problem-solving

Days 11-13: Boundary and agreement establishment

- Create written agreements about household management, decision-making, and communication

- Establish clear consequences for agreement violations

- Practice boundary-setting in daily interactions

- Address areas of chronic conflict with specific behavioral changes

Days 14: Mid-point assessment

- Evaluate progress with professional support

- Adjust strategies based on what's working versus what's still challenging

- Acknowledge improvements while addressing remaining areas of concern

- Recommit to the process or modify goals based on results so far

Week 3: Deepening and integration

Days 15-17: Emotional intimacy building

- Practice vulnerability and emotional sharing without immediate problem-solving
- Create regular time for appreciation and positive focus
- Address sexual or physical intimacy if relevant to relationship concerns
- Build new positive experiences together

Days 18-20: Individual growth focus

- Work on personal issues that contribute to relationship difficulties
- Develop individual interests and support systems
- Practice self-care and stress management techniques
- Support each other's individual therapy or development work

Days 21: Three-week evaluation

- Assess relationship satisfaction improvements
- Identify areas where change feels sustainable versus effortful
- Plan for how to maintain positive changes beyond the 30-day period
- Address any remaining major concerns or obstacles

Week 4: Sustainability planning

Days 22-24: Long-term system development

- Create ongoing maintenance plans for relationship skills

- Establish regular check-in schedules and professional support plans

- Plan for how to handle future stressors and setbacks

- Build accountability systems for continued growth

Days 25-27: Integration with daily life

- Practice new patterns under normal life stress and responsibilities

- Address any remaining areas of conflict or tension

- Plan how new approaches will work with work schedules, parenting, and other demands

- Build confidence in your ability to maintain improvements

Days 28-30: Final evaluation and decision-making

- Comprehensive assessment of relationship changes

- Decision about continuing intensive work, maintaining current improvements, or considering other options

- Celebration of progress made and commitment to continued growth

- Planning for ongoing professional support and skill maintenance

Annual relationship health assessments

Long-term relationship success requires regular evaluation and adjustment of your approaches, goals, and support systems. Annual assessments provide systematic review while preventing problems from building up over time.

Comprehensive relationship evaluation categories:

Communication effectiveness

- How well do we express our needs and concerns to each other?

- Do our conversations typically lead to understanding and resolution?

- Are we able to discuss difficult topics without escalating to conflict?

- How effectively do we handle disagreements and different approaches?

- What communication skills do we want to develop further?

Emotional intimacy and connection

- Do we feel emotionally close and supported by each other?

- Are we comfortable sharing vulnerable feelings and experiences?

- Do we make time for positive, enjoyable interactions?

- How satisfied are we with our level of affection and physical intimacy?

- What would help us feel more connected as a couple?

Individual growth and autonomy

- Are we both continuing to grow and develop as individuals?

- Do we support each other's personal goals and interests?

- Can we maintain our individual identities while building our partnership?

- How well do we balance couple time with independent activities?

- What individual growth would benefit our relationship?

Household and financial management

- How effectively do we share responsibilities and decision-making?

- Are our approaches to money, spending, and financial planning working for both of us?

- Do we feel like equal partners in managing our shared life?

- How well do our different organizational styles complement each other?

- What practical improvements would reduce daily stress?

Parenting partnership (if applicable)

- How well do we support each other's parenting strengths?

- Are we presenting united fronts while respecting different approaches?

- How are our children responding to our relationship dynamic?

- What parenting challenges need our collaborative attention?

- How can we better protect our children from adult relationship stress?

Social and family relationships

- How well do we balance couple time with extended family and friendships?

- Are we supportive of each other's social connections and activities?

- How do our relationships with others affect our partnership?

- What social goals do we have as a couple?

- How can we better integrate our individual social needs?

Future planning and shared goals

- Are we aligned on major life directions and priorities?

- How well do we plan and make decisions about future goals?

- What dreams and aspirations do we want to pursue together?

- How do we balance individual ambitions with partnership goals?

- What shared experiences do we want to create in the coming year?

Annual assessment process:

Preparation phase (2 weeks before assessment)

- Schedule dedicated time for comprehensive review

- Individual reflection on each evaluation category

- Gather any relevant information (financial records, family feedback, etc.)

- Review previous year's goals and commitments

Assessment conversation (2-3 hours)

- Review each category systematically without rushing

- Share individual perspectives and listen to each other's experiences

- Identify areas of satisfaction and areas needing attention

- Avoid problem-solving during assessment—focus on understanding current state

Goal setting session (1-2 hours)

- Choose 3-5 specific areas for focused improvement

- Set measurable, achievable goals for the coming year

- Plan specific strategies and resources for reaching goals

- Establish accountability and review systems

Professional consultation (optional)

- Schedule appointment with couples therapist or relationship coach

- Review assessment results with objective professional guidance

- Get recommendations for resources, strategies, or additional support

- Plan for ongoing professional involvement as needed

Building your permanent support team

Sustainable OCPD relationship management requires ongoing support systems that provide perspective, guidance, and encouragement during both good times and challenging periods. Building this support team is a strategic investment in your relationship's long-term health.

Core support team roles:

Professional therapeutic support Regular individual or couples therapy provides objective guidance, skill development, and crisis intervention when needed.

Choose therapists who:

- Have experience with personality disorders and high-conflict relationships

- Understand OCPD specifically and can provide appropriate strategies

- Support both individual growth and relationship improvement

- Are available for crisis sessions when needed

- Can coordinate with other members of your support team

Medical and psychiatric support Medication management and medical care address any mental health components of relationship challenges.

This might include:

- Psychiatrist for medication evaluation and management

- Primary care physician for stress-related health concerns

- Specialists for any medical conditions that affect relationship stress

- Emergency medical resources for crisis situations

Peer support networks Connections with others who understand OCPD relationship challenges provide validation and practical strategies.

Options include:

- Support groups for partners of people with personality disorders

- Online communities focused on OCPD relationships

- Individual friendships with people who understand your situation

- Couples who have successfully navigated similar challenges

Family and social support Trusted family members and friends who provide emotional support and practical assistance during difficult periods.

Look for people who:

- Understand your commitment to working on your relationship

- Provide support without trying to make decisions for you

- Offer practical help (childcare, meals, etc.) during crisis periods

- Can provide perspective and reality-checking when needed

- Respect your privacy and confidentiality

Professional consultation resources Specialists who can provide guidance on specific aspects of OCPD relationships.

This might include:

- Financial planners who understand relationship dynamics

- Career counselors for individual professional development

- Educational consultants for children's needs

- Legal consultation for understanding your rights and options

Support team coordination:

Clear communication about roles ensures each support person understands how they can best help without overstepping boundaries or creating confusion.

Regular utilization rather than crisis-only contact maintains relationships and prevents support people from feeling used or overwhelmed.

Professional boundaries respect the different roles various support people play rather than expecting friends to provide therapy or therapists to provide friendship.

Coordinated care when multiple professionals are involved ensures they're working together effectively rather than providing conflicting guidance.

Backup plans for when primary support people are unavailable during crisis periods.

Quick reference guides for common scenarios

Having prepared responses for predictable situations reduces stress and improves outcomes when OCPD patterns create relationship challenges.

Scenario 1: Perfectionist episode escalation

What it looks like:

- Partner becomes increasingly anxious about inefficiency or suboptimal outcomes
- Multiple improvement suggestions offered in rapid succession
- Taking over tasks or reorganizing things you've already completed
- Expression of frustration about "chaos" or things being "all wrong"

Your response options:

- "I can see you're feeling anxious about this situation. What would help you feel more comfortable?"
- "I appreciate your suggestions. I'm going to finish this my way, and you can make adjustments if needed."
- "This seems to be triggering perfectionist anxiety. Should we take a break and come back to this later?"

What not to do:

- Argue about whose method is objectively better
- Take their anxiety personally as criticism of your competence
- Try to logic them out of their perfectionist concerns
- Get defensive about your approaches or choices

Scenario 2: Criticism disguised as help

What it looks like:

- "Helpful" suggestions about better ways to do routine tasks

- Detailed explanations of why their approach would produce superior results

- Research presented to demonstrate optimal methods you should adopt

- Expression of concern about your inefficient or suboptimal choices

Your response options:

- "I can see you've found an approach that works well for you. I'm satisfied with my method."

- "Thank you for the information. I'll consider it and let you know if I want to make changes."

- "I appreciate that you want to help. I need space to do this my way."

What not to do:

- Justify your methods or prove they work adequately

- Accept their research as evidence you should change

- Get pulled into debates about efficiency or optimization

- Assume their suggestions mean you're doing something wrong

Scenario 3: Decision-making takeover

What it looks like:

- Partner researches decisions you're making and presents better alternatives

- Pressure to delay choices until more thorough analysis is completed

- Taking over decisions because your approach seems inadequate or risky
- Expression of anxiety about consequences of your less-researched choices

Your response options:

- "I appreciate your research. I'm comfortable making this decision with the information I have."
- "I understand you'd approach this differently. This method works for my priorities and timeline."
- "I can see you're concerned about the outcome. I'm prepared to handle the consequences of my choice."

What not to do:

- Defend your decision-making process as adequate or logical
- Adopt their research requirements to prove you're being responsible
- Delay decisions indefinitely to avoid their anxiety about suboptimal outcomes
- Take responsibility for managing their worry about your choices

Scenario 4: Control through planning

What it looks like:

- Insistence on extensive planning for routine activities
- Detailed research required before making simple choices
- Anxiety about spontaneous activities or unplanned events
- Taking over event planning because your approach isn't thorough enough

Your response options:

- "I appreciate your planning skills. I prefer a more spontaneous approach for this situation."

- "You can plan your activities thoroughly, and I'll handle mine more flexibly."

- "I understand planning reduces your anxiety. I'm comfortable with less structure."

What not to do:

- Argue that extensive planning is unnecessary or excessive

- Try to convince them that spontaneity is more fun or efficient

- Take responsibility for their anxiety about unplanned events

- Abandon all planning to prove your point about flexibility

Scenario 5: Children caught in perfectionist pressure

What it looks like:

- Excessive feedback about children's methods or approaches

- Redoing children's tasks because they don't meet adult standards

- Anxiety about children making mistakes or producing imperfect work

- Pressure on children to optimize their choices or performance

Your response options:

- "I think she's doing age-appropriate work. Let's let her practice her own approach."

- "He's learning, and making mistakes is part of that process."

- "I'm going to step in here so this stays positive for our child."

What not to do:

- Allow perfectionist pressure to overwhelm children's learning process

- Argue with your partner about parenting standards in front of children

- Take over all interactions with children to protect them

- Ignore signs that children are becoming anxious about making mistakes

Emergency contact and resource list

Having easily accessible contact information and resources prevents crisis situations from becoming worse due to inability to quickly find appropriate help.

Immediate crisis resources:

- National Suicide Prevention Lifeline: 988

- Crisis Text Line: Text HOME to 741741

- National Domestic Violence Hotline: 1-800-799-7233

- Local emergency services: 911

- Poison Control: 1-800-222-1222

Mental health emergency resources:

- Local hospital emergency psychiatric services

- Community mental health crisis intervention services

- Your individual therapist's emergency contact information

- Your couples therapist's crisis support information

- Psychiatric medication prescriber's emergency line

Personal support contacts:

- Trusted friend who understands your relationship situation: _____

- Family member who can provide emergency support: _____

- Neighbor or local friend for immediate assistance: _____

- Support group leader or member contact: _____

- Spiritual or religious leader if applicable: _____

Professional service providers:

- Individual therapist: _____

- Couples therapist: _____

- Psychiatrist or medical provider: _____

- Children's therapist or counselor: _____

- Legal consultation if needed: _____

Practical emergency resources:

- Backup childcare for crisis situations: _____

- Safe place to stay if you need to leave home temporarily: _____

- Transportation if your usual methods aren't available: _____

- Financial resources for emergency expenses: _____

- Important documents location: _____

Maintenance planning for long-term success

Sustaining positive changes in OCPD relationships requires ongoing attention and systematic maintenance rather than expecting improvements to continue automatically.

Daily maintenance practices:

- Morning intention setting for how you want to approach relationship interactions

- Mindful communication during routine conversations

- Boundary maintenance in small, daily interactions

- Evening reflection on what went well and what could improve tomorrow

- Self-care practices that maintain your emotional stability

Weekly maintenance practices:

- Relationship check-in meetings using structured format

- Appreciation and gratitude exchanges

- Review of agreements and commitments

- Individual activities that maintain your sense of self

- Connection time that doesn't involve problem-solving

Monthly maintenance practices:

- Assessment of relationship satisfaction and areas needing attention

- Adjustment of agreements or strategies based on what's working

- Professional consultation if patterns are concerning

- Social activities that support your relationship and individual wellbeing

- Planning for upcoming challenges or stressful periods

Quarterly maintenance practices:

- Comprehensive review of relationship goals and progress
- Individual therapy or relationship coaching check-ins
- Assessment of support system effectiveness
- Financial and practical life planning that affects relationship stress
- Celebration of progress and commitment to continued growth

Annual maintenance practices:

- Complete relationship health assessment
- Professional couples therapy intensive or workshop
- Review and updating of emergency plans and support contacts
- Individual and relationship goal setting for coming year
- Vacation or retreat time focused on relationship enjoyment rather than improvement

The emergency toolkit and maintenance plan in this chapter provide comprehensive resources for both crisis management and ongoing relationship health. These systems work because they recognize that OCPD relationships require more intentional management than typical partnerships, while providing hope that this management can become natural and sustainable over time.

Comprehensive resources for ongoing relationship management

The tools and systems outlined in this chapter acknowledge that OCPD relationships benefit from more structure and support than typical partnerships require. This isn't a sign of weakness or failure— it's recognition that personality disorders create ongoing challenges that respond well to systematic approaches.

Having crisis protocols reduces the fear and helplessness that can make temporary setbacks feel devastating. Maintenance plans provide confidence that positive changes can be sustained over time. Support teams offer perspective and assistance that no couple should try to provide entirely for themselves.

Most importantly, these comprehensive resources demonstrate your commitment to creating the best possible outcomes for your relationship, your family, and your individual wellbeing. The time and energy invested in developing these systems pays dividends in reduced crisis frequency, faster recovery from setbacks, and greater overall relationship satisfaction.

Your relationship deserves this level of care and attention. The challenges created by OCPD are real and significant, but they're also manageable with appropriate resources, support, and commitment to ongoing growth and improvement.

Reference

Chapter 1

1. Fineberg, N. A., Sharma, P., Sivakumaran, T., Sahakian, B., & Chamberlain, S. R. (2007). Does obsessive–compulsive personality disorder belong within the obsessive–compulsive spectrum? *CNS Spectrums, 12*(6), 467–482.

2. Hopwood, C. J., Malone, J. C., Ansell, E. B., Sanislow, C. A., Grilo, C. M., McGlashan, T. H., ... Morey, L. C. (2011). Personality assessment in DSM-5: Empirical support for rating severity, style, and traits. *Journal of Personality Disorders, 25*(3), 305–320.

3. Whisman, M. A., & Baucom, D. H. (2012). Intimate relationships and psychopathology. *Clinical Child and Family Psychology Review, 15*(1), 4–13.

Chapter 2

4. Egan, S. J., Wade, T. D., & Shafran, R. (2011). Perfectionism as a transdiagnostic process: A clinical review. *Clinical Psychology Review, 31*(2), 203–212.

5. Pinto, A., Liebowitz, M. R., Foa, E. B., & Simpson, H. B. (2011). Obsessive–compulsive personality disorder as a predictor of exposure and ritual prevention outcome for obsessive–compulsive disorder. *Behaviour Research and Therapy, 49*(8), 453–458.

Chapter 3

6. Clifton, A., Pilkonis, P. A., & McCarty, C. (2007). Social networks in borderline personality disorder. *Journal of Personality Disorders, 21*(4), 434–441.

Chapter 4

7. Bancroft, L. (2015). *Daily wisdom for Why Does He Do That? Readings to empower and encourage women involved with angry and controlling men.* Berkley.

8. Linehan, M. M. (2014). *DBT skills training manual* (2nd ed.). Guilford Press.

9. McKay, M., Wood, J. C., & Brantley, J. (2019). *The dialectical behavior therapy skills workbook* (2nd ed.). New Harbinger.

10. Smith, M. J. (1975). *When I say no, I feel guilty: How to cope—Using the skills of systematic assertive therapy.* Bantam.

Chapter 5

11. Gottman, J. (2011). *The science of trust: Emotional attunement for couples.* W. W. Norton.

12. Johnson, S. M. (2019). *Attachment theory in practice: Emotionally focused therapy (EFT) with individuals, couples, and families.* Guilford Press.

13. Stone, D., Patton, B., & Heen, S. (2010). *Difficult conversations: How to discuss what matters most* (2nd ed.). Penguin Books.

Chapter 6

14. Beck, A. T., Rush, A. J., Shaw, B. F., & Emery, G. (1979). *Cognitive therapy of depression.* Guilford Press.

15. Lavner, J. A., Lamkin, J., Miller, J. D., Campbell, W. K., & Karney, B. R. (2016). Narcissism and newlywed marriage: Partner characteristics and marital trajectories. *Personality Disorders: Theory, Research, and Treatment, 7*(2), 169–179.

16. Neff, K. (2011). *Self-compassion: The proven power of being kind to yourself.* William Morrow.

Chapter 7

17. Flett, G. L., & Hewitt, P. L. (2013). Disguised distress in children and adolescents "flying under the radar": Why psychological problems are underdiagnosed and how schools must respond. *Canadian Journal of School Psychology, 28*(1), 12–27.

18. Morris, L., & Lomax, C. (2014). Assessment, development, and treatment of childhood perfectionism: A systematic review. *Child and Adolescent Mental Health, 19*(4), 225–234.

19. Siegel, D. J., & Hartzell, M. (2003). *Parenting from the inside out.* Tarcher/Perigee.

20. Timpano, K. R., Keough, M. E., Mahaffey, B., Schmidt, N. B., & Abramowitz, J. (2010). Parenting and obsessive–compulsive symptoms: Implications of authoritarian parenting. *Journal of Cognitive Psychotherapy, 24*(3), 151–164.

Chapter 8

21. Ansell, E. B., Pinto, A., Edelen, M. O., Markowitz, J. C., Sanislow, C. A., Yen, S., … Grilo, C. M. (2011). The association of personality disorders with the prospective 7-year course of anxiety disorders. *Psychological Medicine, 41*(5), 1019–1028.

22. Barber, J. P., Morse, J. Q., Krakauer, I. D., Chittams, J., & Crits-Christoph, K. (1997). Change in obsessive–compulsive and avoidant personality disorders following time-limited supportive–expressive therapy: A preliminary report. *Psychotherapy: Theory, Research, Practice, Training, 34*(2), 133–143.

Chapter 9

23. Gottman, J. M. (1999). *The marriage clinic: A scientifically based marital therapy.* W. W. Norton.

24. Johnson, M. P. (2008). *A typology of domestic violence: Intimate terrorism, violent resistance, and situational couple violence.* Northeastern University Press.

25. Karney, B. R., & Bradbury, T. N. (2020). Research on marital satisfaction and stability in the 2010s: Challenging conventional wisdom. *Journal of Marriage and Family, 82*(1), 100–116.

Chapter 10

26. Fisher, H. (2016). *Anatomy of love: A natural history of mating, marriage, and why we stray* (rev. & updated ed.). W. W. Norton.

27. Papp, L. M., Goeke-Morey, M. C., & Cummings, E. M. (2013). Let's talk about sex: A diary investigation of couples' intimacy conflicts in the home. *Couple and Family Psychology: Research and Practice, 2*(1), 60–72.

Chapter 11

28. Panuzio, J., & DiLillo, D. (2010). Physical, psychological, and sexual intimate partner aggression among newlywed couples: Longitudinal prediction of marital satisfaction. *Journal of Family Violence, 25*(7), 689–699.

29. Seligman, M. E. P. (2011). *Learned optimism: How to change your mind and your life.* Vintage.

30. Winnicott, D. W. (1965). *The maturational processes and the facilitating environment.* International Universities Press.

Chapter 12

31. Herman, J. L. (2015). *Trauma and recovery: The aftermath of violence—from domestic abuse to political terror* (updated ed.). Basic Books.

32. Levine, P. A. (2010). *In an unspoken voice: How the body releases trauma and restores goodness.* North Atlantic Books.

33. van der Kolk, B. A. (2014). *The body keeps the score: Brain, mind, and body in the healing of trauma.* Viking.

34. Walker, P. (2013). *Complex PTSD: From surviving to thriving.* Azure Coyote Publishing.

Chapter 13

35. Perel, E. (2006). *Mating in captivity: Unlocking erotic intelligence.* Harper.

36. Schnarch, D. (2009). *Intimacy & desire: Awaken the passion in your relationship.* W. W. Norton.

37. Tatkin, S. (2012). *Wired for love: How understanding your partner's brain and attachment style can help you defuse conflict and build a secure relationship.* New Harbinger.

Chapter 14

38. Bancroft, L., & Silverman, J. G. (2002). *The batterer as parent: Addressing the impact of domestic violence on family dynamics.* Sage.

39. Eddy, B. (2006). *High conflict people in legal disputes.* HCI Press.

40. Johnston, J. R., & Campbell, L. E. (1988). *Impasses of divorce: The dynamics and resolution of family conflict.* Free Press.

41. Lebow, J. (2005). *Handbook of clinical family therapy*. John Wiley & Sons.

Chapter 15

42. Gottman, J. M. (2011). *The science of trust: Emotional attunement for couples*. W. W. Norton.

43. Johnson, S. M. (2008). *Hold me tight: Seven conversations for a lifetime of love*. Little, Brown Spark.

44. Weiner-Davis, M. (2003). *The sex-starved marriage: Boosting your marriage libido*. Free Press. *(Later reprints exist.)*

Chapter 16

45. Karpel, M. A. (1994). *Evaluating couples: A handbook for practitioners*. W. W. Norton & Company.

www.ingramcontent.com/pod-product-compliance
Lightning Source LLC
Chambersburg PA
CBHW060004100426
42740CB00010B/1389